"*Breastfeeding Made Simple* gives mothers the research-based "why" behind every "how." Head reasons for heart feelings! I recommend this groundbreaking book to all my clients and to the people who care about them."

—*Diane Wiessinger, MS, IBCLC*

"*Breastfeeding Made Simple* is fabulous! The research you cite and the ideas you present are so meaningful, yet the whole thing seems very accessible for new moms. I wish I had read this book before I had a baby . . . This book should be a prerequisite for parenting!"

—*Loren, mother of two-year-old Claire, now expecting her second child*

"This book is the most straightforward and informative book about breastfeeding that I've read. I would like to hand out copies to every pregnant woman I see."

—*Kerrie, first-time mother of five-month-old Andrew*

Breastfeeding Made Simple

SEVEN NATURAL LAWS *for* NURSING MOTHERS

NANCY MOHRBACHER, IBCLC

KATHLEEN KENDALL-TACKETT, PH.D., IBCLC

New Harbinger Publications, Inc.

Publisher's Note

This publication is designed to provide accurate and authoritative information in regard to the subject matter covered. It is sold with the understanding that the publisher is not engaged in rendering psychological, financial, legal, or other professional services. If expert assistance or counseling is needed, the services of a competent professional should be sought.

Cover design by Amy Shoup; Acquired by Tesilya Hanauer;
Edited by Carole Honeychurch; Text design by Tracy Marie Carlson

Distributed in Canada by Raincoast Books
All Rights Reserved
Printed in the United States of America

New Harbinger Publications' website address: www.newharbinger.com

FSC

Mixed Sources
Product group from well-managed
forests and other controlled sources

Cert no. SW-COC-002283
www.fsc.org
© 1996 Forest Stewardship Council

Library of Congress Cataloging-in-Publication Data

Mohrbacher, Nancy.
  Breastfeeding made simple : seven natural laws for nursing mothers
  / by Nancy Mohrbacher and Kathleen Kendall-Tackett.
    p. cm.
  Includes bibliographical references.
  ISBN-10 1-57224-404-6
  ISBN-13 978-1-57224-404-7
  1. Breast feeding.   I. Kendall-Tackett, Kathleen. II. Title.
RJ216.M5697 2005
649'.33—dc22
                                    2005022955

11   10   09

15   14   13   12   11   10   9

Contents

■ The Role of History and Culture ■ Commercial Pressures
■ Breastfeeding and the Medical Community ■ Summary

PART II
Applying the Laws

Foreword

How did breastfeeding become so unnecessarily complicated? As the years go by, I am often astounded by how we manage to add new wrinkles of complexity to something that should be easy, natural, and uncomplicated. Of course, breastfeeding itself has not become more complex than it was, say, 200 years ago. Rather, it is the way we think about breastfeeding that has changed.

As a pediatrician working in southern Africa in the early 1980s, I was amazed at how naturally mothers breastfed their babies. They just put the baby to the breast, with no fuss or bother, no diagrams of how the baby should latch on, no concern about how many minutes the baby nursed on each side, no obsession with how many hours between feedings, no anxiety that the baby had fed only six times a day or fourteen times a day instead of the standard North American eight to twelve times, and no one thought that breastfeeding might not work. And again, to my amazement, it almost always did work. The very fact that I was amazed, of course, speaks volumes about what I, brought up and trained as a pediatrician in North America, experienced in my life and professional training. These African mothers, the vast majority of whom had never read a book on breastfeeding, who never attended a prenatal class, who probably couldn't imagine what a lactation consultant would do, seemed to exhibit no more anxiety about how they were breastfeeding than about how they were breathing. Of course, breastfeeding was not always problem free in southern Africa either (just as breathing is not always problem free, if you have asthma, for example), but mothers lived in a culture where breastfeeding was normal, and if mothers did run into problems, they had women all around them (their own mothers, sisters, friends) who had breastfed and who usually knew how to get them through it. In fact, the mothers who seemed to have the most problems were those who were the best educated (in the modern sense) and the most Westernized.

However, this basic, ingrained knowledge of how to breastfeed and care for babies was being lost even in southern Africa by the 1980s, when I was there. More and more mothers were having difficulty with "not enough milk," something that older physicians told me they had never heard of. More were using formula supplements, when their own mothers apparently hadn't needed them years before. Part of the problem was the increasing availability of formula and the allure that formula has for poor people ("I can afford to give my baby formula"), even if they couldn't afford it. An equally important part was the greater availability of Western medicine.

Now, Western medicine has accomplished some pretty marvelous things. Our ability to save the lives of babies born as early as twenty-five weeks or even earlier is nothing less than miraculous and was unheard of even fifty years ago (though the long-term results may not always be as wonderful as we would like). Our ability to treat many kinds of cancer that were previously almost always fatal is another. One thing that Western medicine has not done, however, is produce artificial milk that is the same as human milk. Despite marketing strategies to convince us otherwise, what are commonly called formulas are actually very different from mother's milk.

What happened? Why did women in North America and other affluent areas of the world abandon breastfeeding? By the early 1970s only about 25 percent of all mothers in North America even started out breastfeeding, and most of them had stopped within a few weeks. There were many reasons for this, including the fact that women were returning to outside work shortly after giving birth, as maternity leave was and is virtually nonexistent in the U.S. But equally if not more important was that Western medicine had decided that what human beings made in a factory was better than what had served humanity well for hundreds of thousands of generations. (Many more women are now breastfeeding in the U.S. even though maternity leave is still very short, demonstrating that it is not just outside work that determines breastfeeding rates). How many mothers have come to our breastfeeding clinic, accompanied by their own mothers who told me, "I wanted to breastfeed, but the doctor told me that formula was better"? And this, in the 1960s and 1970s, when formulas weren't as good as they are now (and they're still not up to scratch today and won't be in 2020, either).

When formulas first started to become popular, in the early part of the twentieth century, they were very complicated to make up. Indeed, they were called "formulas" because you took one part of this, another part of that, yet another part of something else, and you had to be very careful to mix the quantities according to the age and size of the baby and their reaction to this milk, which was different than the human milk babies' bodies are designed to eat. The artificial food the baby was drinking was made up from a formula. Furthermore, the immune-deficient, artificially fed baby had to be protected from foreign bacteria, so complicated instructions on how to sterilize the formula and the bottles and the teats were needed. Physicians worked hand in hand with the formula manufacturers to encourage formula use because they suddenly had a new reason for patients to come in. Nursing mothers would never have gone, in those days, to see a physician (almost always men) to ask about breastfeeding issues. They would ask their mothers or sisters. But here was a whole new set of patients, new mothers, who needed to see a doctor to find out how to feed their babies. And with that came information about how to take care of their babies. Rules were needed—otherwise, why would the mother need the doctor? So rules were invented, not only for how to make up formula but also for how often and how long to feed the baby. There were also new rules for child care, rules such as leaving a baby to cry and thus avoiding "spoiling" them by picking them up.

As the years went on, formula preparation became less complicated, with ready-made versions or those that simply needed water added. At the same time, breastfeeding, which had been easy and carefree, became more and more complicated. The rules devised to use in formula preparation and feeding got applied to breastfeeding. After all, when you apply "scientific principles" to feeding an infant with formula it makes sense that breastfeeding should work exactly as formula feeding does. A brief discussion of just a couple of these many rules will illustrate what I mean.

FEED EVERY THREE TO FOUR HOURS

What is it that determines how long a baby should wait between feedings? That's easy—it's the amount of milk they drink. With a bottle, you can force the baby to take more than they really want. If the doctor says the baby should take four ounces, the mother, wishing to obey instructions, tries to make the baby take four ounces, even if the baby really wants only three. This overstuffed child may then sleep three to four hours. With breastfeeding, the baby rarely takes more than they want, and it's impossible to force them to take more. Not only that, with the poor teaching mothers still receive on how breastfeeding works, babies often get less than they'd prefer, even if the milk supply is abundant. If the baby takes only two ounces from the breast, they'll likely wake up in two hours instead of three or four, leading many mothers to conclude that:

- I don't have enough milk.

- Breastmilk is not as good as formula.

- Breastfeeding imposes too many demands on me.

FEED TEN TO TWENTY MINUTES

It takes the average baby about ten to twenty minutes to empty a bottle. Since one bottle is supposed to equal two breasts, the logic says to breastfeed ten to twenty minutes. It seems to make sense, but when you know the differences between the two systems, the analogy is obviously wrong. The breast does not work at all in the same way as the bottle. The bottle gives steady flow throughout the feeding. But the breast gives less flow until the milk release, then more rapid flow than the bottle, and then it slows down again. A mother may have several milk releases during a feeding, so that flow from breast to baby is often up and down. Suggesting that the baby will get 90 percent of the milk in the first ten minutes, as many physicians still do, assumes the breast is like the bottle—but it's not. If the mother believes the ten-to-twenty-minute rule and the baby takes more than this amount of time to feed, the mother may conclude (and may be supported by her doctor):

- I don't have enough milk.

- Human milk is not as good as formula.

- Breastfeeding imposes too many demands on me.

On the other hand, some babies whose mothers have a lot of milk may only feed on one breast for ten or fifteen minutes, or even less, and be perfectly satisfied. But since it takes two breasts to equal one bottle, the mother (and the physician) may conclude:

- The baby is not getting enough milk.

Applying rules that may or may not be appropriate for artificial feeding is obviously not appropriate for breastfeeding. By trying to squeeze a round peg into a square hole, we have twisted and turned our notions of how to breastfeed so that we've lost sight of what breastfeeding is supposed to be like. And mothers are completely stymied by all the conflicting advice they hear, as each health provider gives them a story that best fits with that health provider's notion of how to fit breastfeeding into that square hole. The most consistent thing I hear from mothers coming to our breastfeeding clinic is, "Every nurse and doctor told me something different."

The truth of the matter is that many health professionals have an intrinsic mistrust of nature. We are taught as pediatricians, for example, that a baby is sick unless proved otherwise. This isn't usually said in so many words, but it is the message behind what we do. The fear of litigation plays a large part in this. As pediatricians, we're always assuming the worst, and when you assume the worst, you find easy ways of avoiding it. So, for example, it is obvious that the exclusively breastfed one-day-old baby is getting much less milk than the artificially fed baby. In a bottle-feeding mentality, it is assumed that there is not enough milk in the first few days, before the "milk comes in." But this is taking the bottlefed baby getting artificial milk as the norm. In fact, artificially fed babies are getting too much in the first few days, and this is not necessarily a good thing.

Breastfeeding Made Simple is exactly what the nursing mother needs these days. Learning the natural laws of breastfeeding will help mothers cut through the nonsense that they may hear about breastfeeding from friends, relatives, the media, and, unfortunately, from their health providers. By simplifying breastfeeding, it will work better. By simplifying breastfeeding, mothers and babies will be happier. By simplifying breastfeeding, more mothers will breastfeed more exclusively and longer. This is a book that has long been needed.

—Jack Newman, MD, FRCPC
    Toronto, Ontario
    January 2005

Introduction

Congratulations! You are about to take part in one of life's great miracles—breastfeeding your baby. Despite the fact that some women have a hard time making it work, for the vast majority of women, breastfeeding is entirely possible. It can even be simple, especially if you know the tricks. And we're here to share them with you.

Allow us to introduce ourselves. We are Nancy and Kathy, and between us, we have more than thirty years of experience working with breastfeeding mothers. Nancy breastfed her own three sons, Carl, Peter, and Ben, who are now grown, and she has been working with breastfeeding families since 1982. As a board-certified lactation consultant since 1991, Nancy founded and ran a large lactation private practice in the Chicago area for ten years. She is also the coauthor of the popular *Breastfeeding Answer Book* (2003), a research-based counseling guide used internationally by lactation professionals. Nancy now works as a lactation consultant at Hollister, Incorporated, manufacturer of the Ameda breast pumps, where she talks daily to breastfeeding mothers by phone and provides breastfeeding education to health professionals.

Kathy breastfed her two sons, Ken and Chris, and is a health psychologist and board-certified lactation consultant, and La Leche League leader. She has been working with breastfeeding families since 1994, chairs the New Hampshire Breastfeeding Task Force, and is on the La Leche League International Board of Directors. Kathy is a health researcher at the Family Research Laboratory, University of New Hampshire, and has authored or edited eleven books on a wide variety of topics, including stress and depression in new mothers. Much of Kathy's current work with mothers involves medication use while breastfeeding and the impact of women's emotional health on their breastfeeding experiences. She speaks to audiences of health-care providers on these issues across the country.

In this book, we will share with you the simple dynamics—or "natural laws"—of breastfeeding that all good lactation consultants use to help mothers. If you read this book during pregnancy, you can use these natural laws to avoid breastfeeding problems. If you read this book after your baby's birth, you can use these laws to solve problems and to help meet your breastfeeding goals.

These natural laws are the "secrets" nobody told you about breastfeeding. After generations of bottle feeding, we are now relearning what women used to know about nursing their babies. If you never had the opportunity to see women breastfeed while you were growing up, learning these natural laws is a must. In a world of conflicting information, you can use them to distinguish good breastfeeding advice from bad.

BREASTFEEDING: THE BIOLOGICAL NORM FOR MOTHERS AND BABIES

As we write this book, an advertising campaign promoting breastfeeding has recently finished in the United States. The primary focus of the Ad Council (the company that made the ads) is to promote exclusive breastfeeding for six months. The slogan of the Ad Council's breastfeeding campaign is "Babies were born to be breastfed," meaning that breastfeeding is the biological norm for mothers and babies. Let's take a look at why the Ad Council chose breastfeeding as an important public-health initiative.

Health Outcomes and Human Milk

At this point, the research studies comparing breastfeeding with man-made substitutes number in the thousands, and the findings show striking differences. Researchers have found that during the first year of life, babies fed nonhuman milks have a higher incidence of:

■ Respiratory disease, including pneumonia and bronchitis

■ Diarrhea and other digestive illnesses

■ Ear infections (up to four times more)

■ Urinary tract infections

■ Meningitis

■ Sudden Infant Death Syndrome (AAP 2005)

Babies deprived of human milk's living antibodies are sick more often, have more severe illnesses, and are hospitalized more often and for a longer time (Cunningham et al. 1991). Examining the research worldwide, a 2003 article in the *Lancet* concluded that exclusive breastfeeding for six months could prevent 13 percent of child deaths—or save 1.3 million children annually (Jones et al. 2003). These findings are not confined to the developing world. A 2004 article in *Pediatrics* reported that 21 percent of U.S. infant deaths between one month and one year of age could be prevented if all U.S. babies did *any* amount of breastfeeding (Chen and Rogan 2004). Stated another way, what this really means is that infant formula *increases* U.S. infant deaths during the first year of life by 27 percent. Even more striking, during a baby's first three months, this paper found that exclusive formula feeding *increases infant mortality by 61 percent.*

But the negative health outcomes associated with nonhuman milks are not limited to infancy. Adults who were formula fed as infants have higher incidence of:

■ Allergy

■ Asthma

- Crohn's disease

- Diabetes

- Ulcerative colitis

- Hodgkin's disease

- Leukemia

- Celiac disease

- Childhood cancers

- Breast cancer

- Obesity (AAP 2005; Armstrong and Reilly 2002)

The list of health problems associated with formula continues to grow. In fact, the more we learn, the clearer it becomes that for a baby's immune system to be fully activated after birth, human milk's living antibodies are needed for at least the first twelve months of life.

More Than Food

Your milk is good food for your baby, of course, but it is so much more. At birth, your baby's body expects to receive the unique living components that are in your milk. If your baby is fed nonhuman milks, he will be missing many ingredients essential for normal body function. There are many ways these essential elements affect your baby. You may have read, for example, that formula use has been correlated with lower intelligence (Mortensen et al. 2002). But for now we'll take a close look at the impact of human milk on just two aspects of your baby's body: immune function and digestion.

NORMAL IMMUNE FUNCTION

Let's begin with the role of your early milk, known as *colostrum*, which is in your breasts during pregnancy and after birth. The World Health Organization (2001) calls colostrum "baby's first immunization" because of the many immune factors it contains. These are especially important to your baby during his first weeks outside the protection of your womb, when he is most vulnerable to infection and illness.

Dairy farmers know that the newborn calf deprived of colostrum is a dead calf, because calves are born with little to no inborn protection from illness. What they need in order to survive comes from their mother's colostrum. To protect their newborn calves, farmers move heaven and earth to make sure they get colostrum. We humans receive enough protection from illness and infection before birth to survive without colostrum, as many of us who did not receive colostrum as babies can attest. But although we can live without it, quality of life suffers. A newborn who does not receive his mother's colostrum is a newborn at risk.

Immune factors in both your colostrum and your mature milk (macrophages, leukocytes, secretory IgA, and more) bind microbes and prevent them from entering your baby's delicate tissues. They kill microorganisms and block inflammation. They also promote normal growth of your baby's thymus, an organ devoted solely to developing normal immune function. The thymus in a baby who is fed nonhuman milks is subnormal in size, on average only about half the size of the thymus of an exclusively breastfed baby (Hanson 2004). The immune factors of human milk do not provide breastfed babies an "extra" boost to their immune system. Human milk is the biological norm—what your baby's body needs and expects at birth. The sad reality is that babies who don't breastfeed suffer from immune-system deficiencies (Labbok et al. 2004).

Human milk is even more important to at-risk babies. Premature babies who are formula fed take longer to tolerate oral feedings and are six to twenty times more likely to develop necrotizing enterocolitis, a potentially fatal bowel disease (AAP 2005). Babies born with PKU, a metabolic disorder, lose an average of fourteen I.Q. points if they are fed formula before their disorder is discovered (Riva et al. 1996). Babies born with cystic fibrosis tend to develop symptoms earlier, grow more slowly, and develop more respiratory infections if they are fed any formula at all (Holliday et al. 1991). Babies with cardiac problems have longer hospital stays and have more problems gaining weight if they miss out on mother's milk (Combs and Marino 1993). Bottom line, for a baby's immune system to function normally, he needs mother's milk.

NORMAL DIGESTIVE HEALTH

Human milk also plays a unique role in digestive health. A newborn's digestive system is sterile and immature at birth and needs help in creating the right environment for digestion and normal development. Right from the start, colostrum creates this normal environment in your baby's digestive system by encouraging the growth of the good bacteria (bifidus flora). This good bacteria is responsible for the mild odor of a breastfed baby's stools. A normal gut environment discourages the growth of harmful bacteria and helps a baby's immune system develop properly. If even a small amount of formula or other foods are given, this changes the gut flora so that within twenty-four hours it resembles that of an adult, which is more vulnerable to harmful bacteria and infection. This is one reason why the Ad Council campaign emphasizes exclusive breastfeeding. Once the baby is back to an exclusive human milk diet, it takes two to four weeks for the gut flora to return to normal.

One of the most important functions of colostrum is to seal your newborn's gut to prevent harmful bacteria from sticking to it and penetrating. The junctions between the cells of your baby's intestinal tract are much more open at birth than they will be even several weeks later. While these junctions are open, your baby is vulnerable to allergy triggers (antigens) passing through the gut membranes and causing sensitization. Introducing foreign proteins too early, such as those found in cow's milk and soy-based formulas, can lead to allergy or food intolerance during the first year (Høst 1991).

There are other properties of your milk that are important to your baby's digestive health. For example, growth factors in your milk help your baby's gut to mature more quickly, help the intestinal mucous lining to grow and develop, and strengthen your baby's intestinal barrier. Because a newborn makes few digestive enzymes, human milk provides the bulk of those needed (amylase and bile salts). There are also at least two antioxidants that discourage inflammation (Hanson 2004). All of these components help your baby develop a normal digestive system. Anything less can lead to digestive problems.

ACCEPT NO SUBSTITUTES

Every few years, the formula companies come up with another "new" ingredient to make formula "more like mother's milk." But what they don't tell you is that these vital, living parts of human milk could never survive the canning process, so they will always be missing from formula. Even with the latest new ingredient, there are hundreds of other ingredients in human milk still absent from formula. Some of these science hasn't even identified yet! Our lack of knowledge is reason enough to avoid man-made substitutes unless absolutely necessary. Even without knowing all the components of human milk, the breast-fed baby wins. Breastfeeding is the original no-brainer.

Health Outcomes for You

Our focus up until now has been on your baby. But breastfeeding is also the biological norm for you, and there are negative health outcomes for mothers who don't breastfeed. Moms who don't have greater incidence of postpartum hemorrhage, osteoporosis, and cancers of the breast, uterus, and ovaries (AAP 2005). After birth, mothers who do not breastfeed experience a rapid shift in hormonal levels. Breastfeeding provides a gradual postpartum hormonal shift that can make your transition to motherhood smoother and easier. In chapter 2, we discuss how the hormones of breastfeeding make new motherhood less stressful and bring you and your baby closer. Anything less than exclusive breastfeeding also means a significantly faster return to fertility after birth (AAP 2005).

Breastfeeding can even impact your financial health. Formula costs a minimum of $1200 U.S. during your baby's first year. And depending on the type you use and what your baby can tolerate, it could cost you as much as two to three times that amount. This estimate does not include the cost of feeding equipment and extra health-care costs, as babies on nonhuman milk tend to be sick more often and more severely (Cunningham et al. 1991). If you work outside the home, using formula can mean more days off from work to care for a sick child. Any way you look at it, not breastfeeding is expensive.

We're hoping you find this information motivating. Breastfeeding is much more than a lifestyle choice or a nice "touchy-feely" option. It is well worth it for both you and your baby, even if it's tough at first. When we hear the expression "the best things in life are free," one of the first things that comes to mind for us is breastfeeding.

HOW TO USE THIS BOOK

This book is organized into two parts. The first part explains each of the seven natural laws of breastfeeding and how they work. We will walk with you down the road of normal breastfeeding. Also included in this journey is an explanation of what can happen when the laws are not followed. In chapter 8, we'll also discuss the forces that interfere with the laws and what you can do to counter them.

Part 2 helps you apply the laws to common breastfeeding challenges. It also includes helpful hints on how to fit breastfeeding into your daily life, as well as what to do when normal breastfeeding isn't possible. We include specific information on how to find personal help, as a book can never be a substitute for the one-on-one help of a lactation professional. We also have additional information and resources available on our Web site (www.BreastfeedingMade Simple.com). We will refer you to our site throughout the book.

Regarding our choice of words, we recognize that babies come in two sexes. To acknowledge this while avoiding awkward constructions like "he/she" throughout, we have alternatively referred to babies as "he" or "she" in every other chapter.

Finally, our main purpose for writing this book is to help you meet your breastfeeding goals. To do this, we try to strip away the confusion that often accompanies breastfeeding. By focusing on breastfeeding's most basic principles (rather than a complicated list of "rules"), we hope you will find it easier to relax and enjoy your baby. We want your breastfeeding experience to be as simple and joyful as it was meant to be.

PART I

The Laws

1. Babies Are Hardwired to Breastfeed

2. Mother's Body Is Baby's Natural Habitat

3. Better Feel and Flow Happen in the Comfort Zone

4. More Breastfeeding at First Means More Milk Later

5. Every Breastfeeding Couple Has Its Own Rhythm

6. More Milk Out Equals More Milk Made

7. Children Wean Naturally

CHAPTER 1

Your Baby's Birth

Law 1:   Babies Are Hardwired to Breastfeed

YOUR BABY'S HARDWIRING

We come into a room where a woman is in the last stages of labor. With a final push, the baby is freed from her mother's body. Immediately after she is born, she is placed on her mother's belly. She lies face down and has a chance to get used to the world around her—to breathe on her own, to get used to the louder sounds of the outside world, to adjust to the light. While she is on her mother's belly, she is reassured by her mother's familiar smell and the sound of her voice.

After she has had a while to adjust to the world on the outside, the new baby begins to move purposefully. Pushing with her feet, she slowly moves her way up her mother's body. She travels by her own efforts, slowly but surely toward her mother's breast. She is encouraged by the sound of Mom's voice and by her smell. When the baby reaches her destination, head bobbing, she opens her mouth, attaches to the breast, and begins to suckle.

Newborns' Ability to Self-Attach

This extraordinary ability that newborns possess to move to the breast unaided and attach is something few of us have seen. In a more typical scenario, as soon as the baby is born, she is whisked away by an efficient hospital staff. They immediately clean her, check her, weigh her, and in some hospitals, put drops in her eyes. It is loud and bright and cold. She begins to cry. Welcome to the world!

MAMMALS AND SELF-ATTACHING BEHAVIORS

While the second scenario is more common, the first can occur. When mothers and babies are kept skin to skin in the first hour or two after birth, most healthy babies demonstrate this remarkable ability to move to the breast and self-attach. And this brings us to Law 1: "Babies are hardwired to breastfeed." *Hardwiring* is a term that neuroscientists use to refer to reflexes and instincts that are built in to your baby's body and brain. In terms of Law 1, what this means is that babies are born with reflexes and instincts that urge them on to find and suckle at their mothers' breasts. In this way, human newborns show that they have something in common with mammals of other species. If you have ever watched a mother cat with a litter of kittens, you have seen the little kittens groping along, trying to get next to their mother. Even though they can't see yet, they use their other senses to gravitate toward their mothers and attach to their nipples, where they find food, comfort, and warmth. This instinctual movement is, in fact, essential for their survival. Doesn't it make sense that human babies would also have that capability? And doesn't it make sense for you to take advantage of it?

We'd like to help you use the inborn breastfeeding abilities and behaviors that your baby already has. That your baby has many built-in abilities to help her breastfeed is the good news. The bad news is that these abilities and behaviors can be interrupted, short-circuited, or misinterpreted. Many mothers do not even know they exist. But even if you've gotten off to a rough start, you can use your baby's built-in responses to get back on track.

The Competence of the Newborn

Newborns have some pretty amazing abilities. The work of Dr. Christina Smillie, a pediatrician and board-certified lactation consultant, describes how the calm interaction you have with your baby will allow your baby's amazing abilities to shine through. Diane Wiessinger, MS, IBCLC, a well-known lactation consultant with an academic background in animal biology and behavior, believes that one of the most significant aspects of Dr. Smillie's work is the clues she has discovered to the human version of what is called with other mammals a "feeding sequence." Pick a mammal—any mammal. Now picture a baby of that species being born. What does it do? Marine mammals make their way to the surface, breathe, then find Mama and nurse. Pouched mammals, born so early that their limbs aren't fully developed, wriggle to the pouch, crawl in, and attach to a teat. Foals, lambs, and baby giraffes struggle to their feet and stagger to Mama's udder. Puppies and kittens and piglets all maneuver themselves to a teat. Whatever mammal you chose, we're sure you can picture its babies making their way to their food source (perhaps with some gentle encouragement from Mama) in a feeding sequence that is standard for that species. Not surprisingly, human infants, too, have a feeding sequence. But in humans it is often disrupted by clothing, infant seats, cribs, even by the well-meaning parent who thinks the baby's abrupt tumble from shoulder toward chest is accidental and needs to be halted. The first step in working with your baby's feeding sequence is simply recognizing it for what it is.

HOW YOUR BABY FINDS THE BREAST

A baby's senses play a vital role as she makes her journey to the breast after birth.

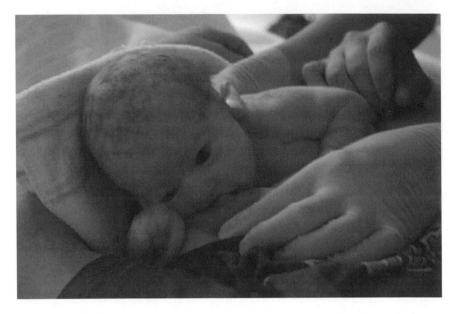

From birth, healthy babies have the amazing ability to make their own way to the breast. (©2005 Prue Carr, used with permission)

Your baby knows your voice, scent, and face. Pediatrician Marshall Klaus and clinical social worker Phyllis Klaus documented in their book, *Your Amazing Newborn* (2000), what your baby can do right after birth. From her first moments, a healthy full-term newborn will make eye contact, will turn toward her mother's voice, and can recognize her mother's scent. Pediatrician and author T. Berry Brazelton found, using his Neonatal Behavior Assessment Scale, that newborn babies will turn toward the sound of their mothers' voices and even prefer that voice to others talking at the same time. Research indicates that newborns find the breast by using their sense of smell, recognize their own mother's voice, respond more distinctly to their own mother's face, and if separated from their mother use a very distinct "separation distress call" to locate her (Bushnell, Sai, and Mullin 1989; Fifer and Moon 1994; Christensson et al. 1995). Your unique scent helps your new baby find you. Her sense of touch (on her chest, cheek, chin, and palate) tells her she is close to the breast. Her body position also tells her when her food source is near. Her senses help orient her toward the breast and help her breastfeed.

The role of hunger and thirst. After the first feeding, biochemistry motivates your baby to self-attach. The first and most obvious biochemical reaction is your baby's level of hunger and thirst. When a baby's blood sugar drops, she starts acting hungry. First, she may awaken from sleep. She puts her hands to her mouth, perhaps chewing or sucking on the back of her hand (Klaus and Klaus 2000). Finally, she will start to cry. As a mother, we encourage you to become aware of your baby's feeding cues, especially the early cues. As we'll discuss in several chapters of this book, it is often difficult to get a screaming baby calmed down enough to breastfeed. And having both of you upset is not an ideal circumstance for you and your baby to learn to breastfeed in the early days.

The role of reflexes. Babies have a stepping reflex that they use to push their way up to the breast after birth. They also root, meaning that when their cheek is touched, they turn toward whatever is touching them (often, the mother's breast) and open their mouths and drop their tongues in anticipation of breastfeeding.

Your baby's responses to the breast. Suckling at the breast calms your baby and can lead to a feeling of fullness. Often, but not always, once a baby feels full, she pulls off the breast and becomes sleepy. Suckling and skin-to-skin contact also release the hormone oxytocin and other substances that relax her. These hormones turn off hunger's stress responses in your baby and promote emotional attachment with you, as we'll describe in chapter 2. Breastfeeding helps your baby connect being close to you with feeling good. The hormones and physical closeness involved in breastfeeding are part of nature's plan to create a strong mother-baby relationship. Mothers and babies can become close without breastfeeding, but it requires more conscious effort.

ARE MOTHERS HARDWIRED, TOO?

While your baby has lots of hardwiring to help her breastfeed, mothers often wonder about themselves. Many mothers ask, "If breastfeeding is so 'natural,' why am I having problems?" After all, cats do it. Mice do it. Even kangaroos do it. Yet in our complex, high-tech world, many human mothers have a hard time making it work.

Maternal Instincts

It's important to clarify what we mean by "instincts." Mothers do indeed come wired with certain predispositions, or tendencies toward specific behaviors. But that does not mean that you will automatically know what to do. When it comes to hardwiring, your baby is actually more instinct-driven than you are.

THE EXTENT OF YOUR HARDWIRING

Your body is designed to respond to your baby. As you hold your baby, your skin temperature goes up or down, depending on your baby's temperature. In other words, your body helps modulate your baby's body temperature. Your nipples are sensitive and become erect to your baby's touch, making locating your breasts easier for your baby.

Breastfeeding releases the hormone oxytocin into your bloodstream, which makes you want to be close to your baby. When your oxytocin levels are elevated, you feel the urge to stroke, touch, and soothe your baby. It also causes your breasts to release milk. As we'll see in chapter 2, oxytocin encourages mothers and babies to be more open to one another and to form close relationships (Uvnäs-Moberg 1998).

THE REST IS LEARNED

Even with all these biological triggers, for mothers, breastfeeding is not instinctive. Although human mothers have biological responses that encourage breastfeeding, they also have free will. Human mothers' instincts are not like those of, say, bees. When bees respond to an instinct, they have no choice but to follow predetermined behaviors. In contrast, humans and some other primates do have a choice. Our bodies may encourage us to behave in a certain way, but we decide whether or not to follow the urge. Our urges can also be overridden by our beliefs or our cultural norms. We'll discuss this effect more in chapter 8.

BREASTFEEDING IS A LEARNED SKILL

The bottom line for you is that while breastfeeding is natural (it's one of the things that makes us mammals), it is also learned. Your body may provide you with cues about what to do. For instance, when you hear your baby cry, your milk may let down. When your baby begins to root or fuss, you may feel a strong urge to pick your baby up and even put her in a position that will allow her to breastfeed, noting that this position seems soothing. But if you haven't seen women breastfeed, you may have no idea what to do next. If this is you, be kind to yourself. Allow yourself the time and opportunity to learn.

When mothers have breastfeeding problems, many admit to either feeling "stupid" or concerned that their maternal instincts are faulty. When mothers share these feelings with us, to put their minds at ease, we often tell the following true story about a gorilla in an Ohio zoo. This gorilla was born in captivity and was not part of a community of gorillas, so she had never seen another gorilla breastfeed. When she gave birth to her first gorilla baby, she had no idea how to feed her and the baby eventually died. When she became pregnant a second time, the zookeepers had an idea. They invited nursing mothers from the local La Leche League group, a mother-to-mother breastfeeding organization, to sit near the gorilla's cage and breastfeed their babies. After watching the human mothers breastfeed, the gorilla mother successfully breastfed her second gorilla baby. Breastfeeding is clearly a learned behavior, even among higher primates.

HOW MOTHERS LEARN TO BREASTFEED

Learning to breastfeed need not be difficult or require lots of instruction. Friends, family, and even health professionals can make breastfeeding sound so complicated that many women worry that they won't be able to do it. This is often a case of too much information given with the wrong emphasis.

Our perspective might strike you as odd, since this is an instructional book about breastfeeding. But stick with us here. Mothers in developed countries have huge amounts of information available on breastfeeding. There are classes, videos, and tons of books. Web sites have a full range of information on everything from common problems to the more obscure. Mothers now have more "expert" information on breastfeeding than ever before.

We are not trying to malign that information in any way. In fact, we've written our share of words about breastfeeding ourselves. But if reading breastfeeding articles or books was enough, the U.S. should have one of the highest breastfeeding rates in the world, which is far from the reality. And in the process, this glut of well-meaning information has managed to make quite a few mothers anxious and confused about breastfeeding.

A different way to think about this is to consider how mothers throughout human history managed to breastfeed without all of the information that we have now. When breastfeeding was the norm, girls learned about breastfeeding as they were growing up by seeing women actually doing it. Dr. Peter Hartmann, a well-known breastfeeding researcher, makes this point well. He asked a young Australian Aboriginal mother, "When did you learn about breastfeeding?" She answered, "I have always known how to breastfeed."

"Head" Knowledge vs. "Body" Knowledge

In Western cultures, we have replaced that kind of "doing" knowledge with book knowledge. And therein lies the challenge. In order to simplify breastfeeding, we want you to understand the built-in mechanisms, or "natural laws," that make breastfeeding easier for you and your baby. In the process, we also want to avoid giving you lots of left-brained "head" knowledge about breastfeeding.

Using Dr. Smillie's term, we prefer to think of breastfeeding as a "right-brained activity." What do we mean by that? Think of left-brained instructions as head knowledge. Right-brained learning yields heart or body knowledge. To illustrate this difference, think about riding a bike. Did you learn by reading about it? Taking a class? Talking to other people about it? Or did you learn by just getting on a bike and doing it?

Learning a second language is another example. Studies with children and adults have found that those who learn a second language like they've learned a first language (by just jumping in and speaking) are much more likely to attain fluency than those who learn mostly in the classroom. Case in point, someone we know named Kate plodded her way through four years of high-school German. Her best friend, Annette, took these classes with her but had the added advantage of growing up in a German-speaking home. Kate did better on grammar and vocabulary tests, but Annette could actually speak the language with near fluency. These really are two entirely different sets of skills. Which would you prefer to be able to do? Language learning is an apt comparison because it is also a human drive—humans will learn to speak unless there are dire circumstances (such as severe abuse or neglect) that prevent this process from happening.

The Right-Brained Dance of Breastfeeding

Mothers are influenced in many ways. Mothers and babies have physiological responses that draw them to each other, that encourage them to look at each other, touch each other, and interact. Much of this behavior is guided by the right side of the brain. This is the side that has to do with affect or emotion. In fact, some characterize mothers' and babies' interactions as an affective "dance," in which the actions of one influence the actions of the other.

How Overthinking Breastfeeding Can Hinder You

A problem with the heavily left-brained, instructionally oriented way that many mothers learn to breastfeed is that it doesn't allow mother and baby to take advantage of their natural responses (Smillie 2004). So much breastfeeding education focuses on all the things the mother must do to get the baby to breastfeed, which ignores the baby's role. That type of instruction can be helpful to solve a particular problem, but it can be a definite drawback when one technique or strategy is applied to all mothers, a "one-size-fits-all" approach to breastfeeding. It also discourages mothers and babies from using their hardwiring. Worse still, this kind of education can encourage them to tune out their natural responses or to violate their instincts. It can be upsetting for all who are involved, sometimes creating a crisis where none existed before.

Another problem with highly instructionalized left-brained approaches is that they can leave some mothers feeling incompetent, because it feels as if there is a list of ten thousand things they need to remember.

Breastfeeding the Right-Brained Way

Now let's get more specific. How exactly do you use a right-brained approach to breastfeed your baby?

BREASTFEEDING AS A RELATIONSHIP

First, take some deep breaths and let go of those worries about doing things "wrong." Instead of thinking of breastfeeding as a skill you need to master, or a measure of your worth as a mother, think about breastfeeding as primarily a relationship. As you spend time with your baby, you'll be more adept at reading her cues. As you hold her (and we encourage you to hold your baby a lot), your baby will be more comfortable in seeking your breast. Breastfeeding will flow naturally out of your affectionate relationship. Based on her extensive clinical experience with mothers and babies, pediatrician and board-certified lactation consultant Christina Smillie has developed some strategies that can help you help your baby. Here are some specific things you can do.

Start with a calm, alert baby. One mistake that many women make is to wait to try breastfeeding until their babies are either sound asleep or screaming. Think about yourself. Do you learn best when you are asleep or upset? Probably not.

There's another reason to start with a calm baby. This one is based on pure physics. When your baby is crying, note where her tongue is. In most cases, it is on the roof of her mouth—unless she is lowering it to take a deep breath before screaming again. If her tongue is raised, how is she going to get your breast in her mouth? The quiet, alert state is when your baby is in the best frame of mind to both learn and to feed.

Watch for early feeding cues. These cues include rooting (turning her head when something touches her cheek) or hand-to-mouth (see chapter 4 for more on this.) It's obviously better if you can catch your calm, alert baby at the first sign of hunger. Take note of when she starts smacking her lips or putting her hands to her mouth. This is an ideal time to try breastfeeding.

Sometimes you don't catch your baby in the early hunger stages (such as when you're sound asleep!) and have to deal with a baby who is upset. And some babies go from a little hungry to very hungry in a really short time. To calm your baby, offer the breast. If this doesn't work, don't force the issue or you'll end up with a real problem, like a baby who associates her time at the breast with frustration. Try these suggestions instead.

Use your body to calm your baby. One way to calm a crying baby is by placing your baby skin to skin vertically between your breasts. That means stripping your baby down to her diaper and either wearing a roomy shirt that can cover you both, or in the privacy of your own home, simply not wearing anything on top. Your chest is a very calming place for your baby (Smillie 2004). She can hear your voice and your heartbeat. She can smell you and get the feeling of your skin. You can also try lifting your baby to your shoulder, patting her back, rocking her, or walking with her. Try talking with her and making eye contact. All of these activities can get her to calm down, allowing your baby to seek the breast on her own.

Follow your baby's lead. When a calm, alert baby is held vertically between her mother's breasts, often she will begin showing instinctive breast-seeking behaviors, bobbing her head and moving it from side to side. Once your baby starts these behaviors, help her in her efforts. Following the baby's lead, support her head and shoulders. Move her rump toward your opposite breast. Encourage her explorations with your voice (Smillie 2004). Babies can't understand your words at this age, but they can understand your tone of voice. When a baby hears a calm, encouraging voice, she feel emboldened to try new things. Help your baby into a horizontal position. Use the other tips listed below and in chapter 3 to help use her hardwiring to latch on to the breast with a minimum of frustration.

Play while you learn to breastfeed. Play is something that is largely absent in the mothers that we see. Often, especially if they are having problems, the mothers are distraught, worried about doing things wrong, and feeling like they are failing this first "crucial test" of motherhood. If you're feeling frustrated, we'd like to encourage you to look at this another way. Focus on your relationship with your baby and consider breastfeeding as a part of this larger whole. As we described earlier, breastfeeding will flow naturally out of your affectionate relationship.

For instance, your baby may try to latch on when not particularly hungry, but when she is trying out her new skill. These practice times are good for your relationship and will serve you well when she is hungry (Smillie 2004).

Can you see how this approach differs from one that emphasizes only picking up your baby when she is screaming or seeing your baby as a blank slate who relies on you to do everything right? Having worked with lots of mothers and babies over the years, we've always been amazed at how well breastfeeding can work when mothers and babies are ready and responsive to each other.

USING OTHER ASPECTS OF YOUR BABY'S HARDWIRING

When we say that babies are hardwired to breastfeed (Law 1), we mean that they are born with natural reflexes that help them find and suckle at their mothers' breasts. This includes the instinctive drive to find your breasts, as we discussed earlier. Here are some other ways you can take advantage of your baby's hardwiring.

Make sure baby's body is not twisted, and close any gaps between you. Hold your baby close from head to toe, with your baby's head, neck, and shoulders in a straight line. Make sure that her body is not twisted. No matter what position you use during feedings, she will feel more secure and relaxed if she feels your steadying warmth against her whole body. Holding your baby skin to skin is even better (see chapter 2 for more). If there are large enough gaps between you and your baby to allow her to pull up her legs, latching on will be more difficult. If the bottom of her feet come in contact with a firm surface, her natural response will be to push away, which also can lead to frustration. To avoid these challenges, pull your baby's whole body firmly against you.

Snuggle your baby's chest and shoulders in tight. When you are ready for her to latch on, pull your baby's chest and shoulders firmly against you. Having her chest and shoulders held stably against your body makes it easier for her to coordinate her head and neck movements during latch-on. A baby whose chest and shoulders are *not* in firm contact with her mother during latch-on can feel as insecure as a ballerina on a moving stage (Glover 2004) and may easily become frustrated. We have personally found the following strategy helpful when working with mothers.

A light touch to trigger a wide-open mouth. For a good, deep latch-on, babies need to open wide while attaching to the breast, and your baby's hardwiring can help with this. (We'll describe this more in chapter 3.) To help your baby open wide, use a repeated light touch of your breast against her chin and lips. By helping your baby move toward and away from the breast, touching it lightly, she will feel the cue she is looking for and will know to open really wide ("wait for the gape" is an expression used in many parts of the world). When a baby feels this touch, it's as though you are speaking her language. And remember, it's fine to experiment, as there is more than one right way to do this. The more you do what works for both you and your baby, the easier and more automatic breastfeeding will become.

The drinking position: Head back, chin forward. Rebecca Glover RM, IBCLC (2002), a midwife and lactation consultant from Australia, notes another aspect to babies' hardwiring. When babies get ready to feed, they instinctively throw their head back and thrust their chin forward. She points out that we adults also do this when we're thirsty and drink fast (think about how you chug a tall, cool glass of water on a hot day).

To understand why babies do this, put your chin to your chest and try to swallow. See how difficult that is? To keep your throat open for drinking, it works best to have your head slightly tilted back. It's the same for babies. However you hold your baby at the breast, be sure she can tilt her head slightly back into this instinctive feeding position. This will make drinking much easier for her.

Feeling the breast in the comfort zone. This point is covered in detail in chapter 3 but deserves a mention here. There is a special place deep in your baby's mouth that triggers active sucking. When you achieve a deep latch and your nipple reaches this "comfort zone," not only is breastfeeding comfortable for you, but your baby's hardwiring is triggered to help her feed well and actively. When she feels your breast there, she gets a better milk flow and breastfeeding is easier. A shallower latch results in a slower milk flow, which can cause many babies to fall asleep quickly and "tune out" at the breast.

Keep mother and baby skin to skin. If you are reading this during your pregnancy, make arrangements to stay skin to skin with your baby for that first hour or two after birth if at all possible. This is one of the easiest ways to trigger your baby's hardwiring. Because you will probably not be in a state of mind to take charge right after giving birth, it is best to arrange for your partner or labor support person to be responsible for talking to the staff about your wishes. If you and your baby are healthy, the birth staff should be expected to honor this request, even if they are unfamiliar with babies' instinctive behaviors. This is one easy and effective way to help get breastfeeding off to a good start.

Using your baby's hardwiring, especially when you're skin to skin (see the next chapter), will help you tune in to your baby's cues more easily. You will spend more time touching, stroking, and talking to your baby, which helps her neurological development and increases your milk supply. With practice, you will begin to feel like the real expert on your baby. And it will help you see your baby as competent, too. You won't need outside experts to tell you that you're doing a good job, because you'll be able to see it with your own eyes. And watching your baby thrive is the best part of all.

WHEN THE SYSTEM BREAKS DOWN

Babies are born knowing how to make their way to the breast, but there are factors that can interfere with this natural process. Knowing this can help you get a good start.

Birth Interventions and Separation

Research has found some of the choices made during and after birth can affect your baby's self-attaching behaviors. In one study of eighty mothers and babies, two factors were found to short-circuit, at least temporarily, a baby's urge to self-attach:

■   The use of Demerol, a narcotic pain reliever, during labor.

■   A short separation of mother and baby for cleaning and weighing before the first breastfeeding.

Not one of the babies who experienced both of these factors attached to the breast and breastfed well during the first two hours after birth. Of the babies who experienced only one of these factors, about half breastfed well in their first two hours. Of the babies who experienced neither—no separation after birth and no Demerol during labor—all breastfed well during this time (Righard and Alade 1990).

Because birth is tiring for both you and your baby, after this first two hours most babies go into a long stretch of sleep. Missing this first feeding decreases the number of total breastfeedings you can fit in during the first twenty-four hours. The overall number of breastfeedings this first day can affect how long it takes for your milk to increase and whether or not your baby develops exaggerated newborn jaundice (see chapter 4). Missing this first feeding is definitely not enough to compromise breastfeeding (legions of mothers and babies whose first breastfeeding was delayed can attest to this), but it puts you and your baby at higher risk for problems and complications. By setting up the right conditions during these first two hours and encouraging self-attaching behaviors after birth, this first law can help you avoid potential problems down the line.

Also, it's important to know that this is not the only study that has found that labor medications and birth interventions can affect breastfeeding. One study found an association between the use of several pain medications given to mothers in labor with more crying, a decrease in breast-seeking behaviors, and less suckling in their newborns (Ransjö-Arvidson et al. 2001). Another study found that the babies of mothers who received an epidural during labor were less alert, less able to orient themselves, and had less organized movements as compared with babies whose mothers received no pain medication during labor (Sepkoski et al. 1992). Surprisingly, researchers found that these differences continued throughout the babies' first month of life.

Birth interventions, such as roughly sucking the mucus from the nose and mouth and the use of forceps or vacuum extraction, can also affect a baby's willingness to breastfeed after birth. And although it is beyond the scope of this book to comprehensively cover the effects of birth interventions on breastfeeding, we encourage you to learn more.

To this end, we recommend the book *Impact of Birthing Practices on Breastfeeding* (2004) by Mary Kroeger with Linda J. Smith, which is listed in our Resources section at the end of this book.

Hospital Routines

Many of the routines followed in hospitals today were created during a time when formula feeding was the norm. From the hospital's standpoint, it made no sense to keep mothers and babies together when most babies were fed nonhuman milks. On the contrary, the focus was on helping the mother to "get her rest," and limiting her contact with her baby was central to that.

GETTING YOUR REST

The issue of getting your rest is obviously legitimate, especially after a long or difficult labor. But no one should ever have to choose between getting her rest and feeding her baby! In breastfeeding-friendly hospitals, mothers are helped to get their rest while they breastfeed. In one hospital in central Illinois, the lactation consultant trains the staff nurses to help mothers feed their babies while lying down. This allows mothers to nap and feed at the same time. One study, not surprisingly, found that women who breastfeed lying down report less fatigue than women who breastfeed sitting up (Milligan et al. 1996).

TASK FOCUS VS. HUMAN NEEDS

In some institutions, mother-baby separation and "sanitary procedures" are still considered more important than a mother and her baby getting to know each other. Sometimes this process is interrupted for no other reason than that the mother and baby are not conforming to the hospital's sense of time. Perhaps the hospital staff needs the room for another mother. Or maybe allowing the mother and baby to just "be" doesn't appeal to the hospital staff's sense of aesthetics or efficiency. In these cases, the justification doesn't really hold up. As we mentioned earlier, when the baby is immediately whisked away to be cleaned, measured, etc., that quiet receptive period after birth is lost. When mother and baby are separated after birth and before the first feeding, babies' ability to self-attach can be sabotaged or suppressed, making breastfeeding more difficult.

Medical Condition of the Mother or Baby

Sometimes mothers or babies are not able to start breastfeeding right away because one or both of them have a medical condition that needs to be attended to immediately. The mother and baby's health take precedence over getting to know each other. For example, if a mother is hemorrhaging, she needs immediate attention. If a baby isn't breathing or has some other emergency medical issue, that needs to be dealt with at once.

Some mothers who have had surgical births may also be separated from their babies immediately after birth. However, in many hospitals, mothers are helped to breastfeed right after a cesarean birth, while they are still comfortable and before their pain medication wears off.

If You Get Off to a Difficult Start

If you have somehow gotten off to a bad start, for whatever reason, do not fear. Baby's instinctive breast-seeking behaviors don't disappear immediately after birth, and you can continue using them to make breastfeeding work. Dr. Christina Smillie has found through her practice that several months after birth, even if the baby hasn't been breastfeeding or feeding well, in healthy babies these instinctive behaviors remain intact. This is great news for mothers and babies who've gotten a rocky start.

IS IT TOO LATE?

We are grateful for the pioneering work of Marshall Klaus and John Kennell in the study of mother/infant bonding and the importance of that time immediately after birth. Unfortunately, in actual practice, we've seen this research badly applied. Some mothers truly believe that if they miss that initial time (as many do), then all is lost. This was never supposed to be the message of the bonding research! It's true that the contact immediately after birth can make things easier. However, breastfeeding and bonding with your baby are too critical to your baby's well-being to be given only one chance to work. The good news is that even if you missed that early time together, it is definitely not too late (Smillie 2004). Babies still know how to self-attach. This ability is not limited to the first twenty-four hours after birth. You can help your baby use this amazing ability through your physical closeness with each other and your playful interactions. These will help your baby breastfeed like the competent little being she is.

CHAPTER 2

The Power of Skin-to-Skin

Law 2: Mother's Body Is Baby's Natural Habitat

WHY SKIN-TO-SKIN FEELS RIGHT

There's nothing that feels quite so right as a mother holding her baby skin to skin. A baby's smell and the feel of a baby's skin are intoxicating. For a baby, too, there is nothing as comforting as his mother's touch. Yet, as universal and as human as these feelings are, there is more to it than that. Much more.

That mothers love to touch their babies is nothing new. What *is* new is our increasing understanding of the power of touch. In fact, in some parts of the world and in some situations, the simple act of a mother holding her baby close has made the difference between life and death.

Lactation consultants and other skilled breastfeeding counselors have long known that putting mothers and babies skin to skin helps solve breastfeeding problems. But now we are beginning to learn why. And the story is a fascinating one.

The Habitat of the Human Newborn

To begin to understand the power of skin-to-skin contact, we must take you on an excursion through mammalian biology. To do this, we draw upon the work of Dr. Nils Bergman, a South African pediatrician who has had remarkable success in decreasing infant mortality in rural Zimbabwe, a part of the world that lacks incubators and other technology found in most hospital special-care nurseries (2001). By wrapping tiny premature babies skin to skin with their mother twenty-four hours a day, which he calls "Kangaroo Mother Care," Dr. Bergman used the power of skin-to-skin to improve infant survival of the smallest preemies in Zimbabwe from 10 percent to a remarkable 50 percent (Bergman and Jurisoo 1994). In the process, we have learned much about the power of skin-to-skin contact, not just as it benefits preemies, but also as a way to promote normal health and breastfeeding for full-term, healthy newborns.

Dr. Bergman is not only a medical doctor; he also has an interest in animal biology and behavior, and his studies into other species were instrumental in the development of his Kangaroo Mother Care approach. In fact, he uses the biologist's term "habitat" to explain why Kangaroo Mother Care has saved so many babies' lives. *Habitat* is the place where behavior occurs. And the mother's body is a baby's natural habitat, the place where babies breastfeed.

All mammals have behaviors that are programmed into their hardwiring and vary depending on their habitat or location. Dr. Bergman (2001) points out: "Mothers don't breastfeed. *Babies* breastfeed. The mother's body is simply the habitat where the baby feeds." It is best to keep mother and baby together right from birth. As we discussed in chapter 1, if a baby is left on his mother's abdomen after a medication-free birth, the newborn, without help from anyone, makes his way to the breast, finds the nipple, and starts breastfeeding. He responds to his mother's scent, her voice, and the feel of her skin. For human infants, breastfeeding and being held close to mother arecritical to survival. The behavior, in this case breastfeeding, is determined by the habitat—baby's closeness to his mother's body.

A Newborn Mammal's Natural Programming

If a newborn is removed from his habitat, his mother's body, it triggers instincts that can be counterproductive to breastfeeding. Dr. Bergman explains that in all mammal babies, there are two basic "programs" governed by the part of the brain called the "hindbrain." These two programs, defense and nutrition, are keys to our survival. They regulate hormones, nerves, and muscles, and affect the whole body. The problem is that at any given time only one program can run. If the defense program is running, the body shuts off the nutrition program, and with it, growth. If the nutrition program is running, a baby's defenses are shut down.

Separation, the defense program, and the protest-despair response. For a newborn, separation from his mother throws his body into defense mode. If you separate a human baby (or any other mammal) from his mother, a physical reaction occurs and the baby responds by loudly protesting with a distinctive cry known as the "separation distress call" (Christensson et al. 1995). Biologists call the set of behaviors that occur when babies are removed from their mothers the "protest-despair response."

When a baby's protest is prolonged and unanswered, the next emotion he experiences is despair. Once this programming has been triggered, a baby goes into defense mode, and to increase the odds of survival, his body shuts down to use less energy by decreasing his heart rate, breathing rate, and body temperature. In this mode, every other function is shut down so that no growth is taking place.

When a baby is in the protest phase, his tiny body produces huge amounts of stress hormones, and the baby physically prepares to fight for survival. This is a baby's version of the "fight-or-flight" response. The stress hormones shut down gut function, digestion, and growth. In fact, Dr. Bergman points out that what is now considered by many medical experts to be the normal ranges of heart rate, body temperature, and stress hormones of preemies separated from their mothers in high-tech nurseries is not normal at all but reflects this protest-despair response. Interestingly, this same reaction occurs in every mammal that's ever been studied.

If you've ever wondered why some babies have such a hard time being set down and left alone, now you know. A newborn's whole body is set to react intensely to separation from his mother. Considering that a newborn's inborn programming is still set as if he were born during caveman times (when separation meant death), this could be considered a survival mechanism.

The nutrition program promotes growth. In contrast, when a newborn is held skin to skin with his mother, the opposite reaction occurs. Being in his natural habitat (touching his mother's body) stimulates the nutrition program. As Dr. Bergman describes (and as his amazing results with premature babies have demonstrated), when a newborn is in the right habitat (touching his mother), his brain responds by triggering the program for growth. His level of stress hormones decreases by 74 percent. His gut begins to process food (Urnäs-Moberg et al. 1987). His heart rate and breathing return to normal. If the baby is in skin-to-skin contact with his mother, he can more easily care for himself.

Not surprisingly, other primates also have a strong drive to be in snuggle-contact with their mothers. Nearly fifty years ago, Harry Harlow conducted a series of experiments in which newborn monkeys had access to both a wire mesh "mother" and a terry-cloth "mother" (Harlow 1959). In some cages one mother had an attached bottle, in other cages, not. No matter which mother provided food, babies spent far more time cuddling on the cloth mother than on the wire mesh mother. Harlow noted that when baby monkeys had no access to a cloth mother, they developed strong attachments to the cloths that lined their cage in ways that reminded him strongly of human childhood attachments to blankets and teddies. Without anything soft to cling to at all, baby monkeys became emotionally disturbed and had difficulty surviving. He noted, "We were impressed by the possibility that, above and beyond the bubbling fountain of breast or bottle, contact comfort might be a very important variable in the development of the infant's affection for the mother" (Harlow 1959, p. 577).

THE EFFECTS OF SKIN-TO-SKIN CONTACT AFTER BIRTH

In light of these remarkable differences in programming, is it any wonder that skin-to-skin contact between mother and baby helps to promote breastfeeding? All of these findings explain why putting baby back into his natural habitat calms and normalizes his nervous system, making him more receptive to growth-promoting behaviors such as feeding and digestion.

Much research has confirmed the positive effects of skin-to-skin for premature babies. But there is also interesting research on its effect on full-term healthy babies. These studies indicate that babies who are kept skin to skin with their mothers for the first couple of hours after birth:

- are more likely to latch on and breastfeed (Righard and Alade 1990);

- are more likely to breastfeed well (Righard and Alade 1992);

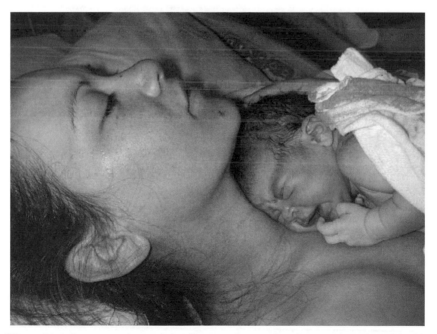

Skin-to-skin calms you and your baby. Your touch is vital to his growth and good health. (©2005 Marilyn Nolt, used with permission)

- cry up to ten times less (Michelsson et al. 1996; Christensson et al. 1995);

- have more stable temperature and higher blood sugar (Christensson et al. 1992), which reflect healthier, more stable body function.

Early skin-to-skin contact between mother and baby has also been found to affect how long mothers and babies breastfeed, with more skin-to-skin contact after birth linked to increased breastfeeding duration (Mikiel-Kostyra, Mazur, and Boltruszko 2002).

HOW SKIN-TO-SKIN WORKS

Science has proven that skin-to-skin contact between mother and baby has profound effects on them both. Now let's take a closer look at the reasons.

If It Feels Good, Oxytocin Must Be Involved

There is far more to our mental and emotional states than just our hormones. But we also know that our hormones can affect us, sometimes in subtle ways. *Oxytocin,* which comes from the Latin word meaning "swift birth," is both a hormone and a central nervous system neurotransmitter and is released during skin-to-skin contact.

THE ROLES OF OXYTOCIN

Oxytocin has a role in many aspects of human physiology, many of which affect relationships. If you are unfamiliar with oxytocin, here are some examples of when it is released and what it does:

- It is released during orgasm in both men and women.

- It causes the contractions of the uterus during labor (its synthetic form, pitocin, is sometimes given to induce or speed labor) and during breastfeeding.

- It is released when a person experiences warm temperatures, touch, stroking, acupuncture, and massage.

- It is directly responsible for milk release, or "letdown," during breastfeeding (Newton 1978).

Scientists have been studying oxytocin for many decades, and some of their findings explain why skin-to-skin contact has such far-reaching implications to biology and behavior. For example, physical effects of oxytocin and related peptides include:

- greater blood flow to the breasts in mothers and to the skin of infants;

- increased appetite and greater digestive efficiency;

- decreased blood pressure and production of stress hormones, such as cortisol;

- increased blood sugar and insulin levels;

- increased pain threshold and enhanced wound healing.

One interesting property of oxytocin is that, although its direct effect on the body is only minutes long, its long-term effects can last for weeks (Uvnäs-Moberg 1998). Oxytocin produces physical changes that have also been found to affect mood and behavior. It has a sedating effect, calms mood, and increases stable personality traits. It decreases the desire to move around and increases the tolerance of monotony. It increases openness to social direction and bonding with peers. It increases "nesting" behaviors. And it enhances acceptance of offspring and bonding between mother and baby. From what we know, oxytocin appears to play a key role in bringing people together and cementing relationships (Uvnäs-Moberg 1998).

Oxytocin and milk release. During breastfeeding, oxytocin is responsible for the release of milk from the breast (sometimes called the "letdown" or "milk-ejection reflex"), a vital aspect of successful breastfeeding and milk expression. Many women think that milk flow from the breast (either to the baby or to a pump) occurs as a result of suction. Actually, that is not the case. Getting milk from the breast is not like sucking liquid through a straw. With a straw, the stronger you suck, the more liquid you get. With the breast, however, strength of suction has little to do with effective breastfeeding or pumping (Mitoulas et al. 2002). The key to milk flow is triggering a milk release.

When a baby latches on to the breast and begins to suckle, the nerve impulses sent to the mother's brain cause the release of oxytocin in her bloodstream. As in labor, oxytocin causes muscles to contract. But the muscles responsible for milk release are in the breasts. These muscles squeeze the milk-producing glands and actively push the milk toward the nipple while the milk ducts widen. Some mothers feel this as a tingling sensation in their breasts; others feel nothing. Some women leak milk from the other breast when the milk releases; others don't. When you hear your baby swallowing, you know you've had a milk release. A milk release can be triggered by many things: a certain touch at the breast, hearing a baby cry, or even by thinking about your baby. Feelings of tension, anger, or frustration can block it.

During breastfeeding, most mothers have several milk releases without even knowing it (Ramsay et al. 2004). The physical cues from your baby make milk release happen automatically. Your baby is soft; your baby is warm; you love your baby. All of these cause your milk to flow. When a mother pumps, these physical cues are missing, so getting a milk release can sometimes be trickier, but there are ways to make this happen. For more on this, see chapter 9.

Breastfeeding lowers stress levels. Some mothers are told by the uninformed that breastfeeding is stressful. Of course, breastfeeding problems can be stressful. But if breastfeeding is going smoothly, actually, the opposite is true. While caring for a newborn can most definitely be intense and sometimes stressful (no matter how he is fed), this is unrelated to breastfeeding.

Considering what we know about oxytocin, it's not surprising that research indicates *not breastfeeding* is more stressful than breastfeeding. The extra time spent skin to skin and the subsequent oxytocin release that is a normal part of breastfeeding no doubt play a part in this. One recent study of a group of women who breastfed *and* bottle-fed demonstrates the calming effect of breastfeeding. Researchers assessed the study mothers' mood before and after breastfeeding and before and after bottlefeeding. Their findings indicated that the study mothers were calmer after breastfeeding than after bottlefeeding. This study was significant because it eliminated one of the major problems in comparing breastfeeding and non-breastfeeding women: the often substantial differences between women who choose one feeding method over the other. Since the same mothers were studied after both breast and bottle, this potentially confounding factor was eliminated (Mezzacappa and Katkin 2002).

THE HORMONE OF LOVE

Oxytocin is sometimes called "the hormone of love." Whenever pleasure is involved, oxytocin appears to be at work. But there is much more to it.

Tend and befriend. Psychologist Shelly Taylor, Ph.D., and her colleagues put forth an intriguing theory stating that males and females respond to stress differently. Because the well-known fight-or-flight response to threat was based mostly on studies of males, they argue that it does not accurately describe the females' response. After all, for females, fighting or fleeing could compromise the survival of their off-spring. Instead, these researchers hypothesized that females respond to stress by tending to their offspring and that this response lowers their overall stress level. One study they cite that supports their theory found that when women had a stressful day at the office, they were more affectionate and nurturing with their children once they got home. The same pattern did not appear for males who tended to withdraw. There does seem to be a limit to this effect though, because when mothers were chronically stressed, they also tended to withdraw from their children, acting more like the males in the study (Repetti, 1997 cited in Taylor et al. 2000). The researchers speculated that the release of oxytocin may be the biobehavioral link to both stress reduction and caregiving behavior.

The "befriend" part of the tend-and-befriend response refers to the tendency of females to seek relationships with other females when under stress. The researchers noted that some of these behaviors could lead to increased survival of offspring for animals and humans. Befriending other females by joining social groups and networks relieves stress, offers protection, and may mean shared childcare. Oxytocin (as well as other substances such as endorphins and estrogen) appears to encourage these behaviors and foster a caregiving and friend-seeking response to stress.

Effects on you. The oxytocin response triggered by both skin-to-skin and breastfeeding has the potential for many far-reaching effects on you. It causes a decrease in aggressive and defensive feelings, making you feel more open to the new little "stranger" to whom you have given birth. Oxytocin influences your mood, makes you calmer, and promotes a closer relationship with your baby and your partner. The effects of oxytocin may also help with relationships outside your family. This may be one reason why many breastfeeding mothers love the atmosphere of mothers' groups, where those with high levels of oxytocin gather to tend and befriend one another.

Mothers of premature babies have found some special benefits to skin-to-skin contact with their babies via Kangaroo Mother Care. In one study of mothers of hospitalized preemies, skin-to-skin contact between mother and baby was positively correlated to more milk pumped (Hurst et al. 1997). In one published case study, skin-to-skin contact with her preemie was considered key in helping a mother with a history of past abuse, depression, and substance abuse make a positive transition to motherhood (Dombrowski, Anderson, and Santori 2001).

Effects on your baby. Skin-to-skin contact, stroking, and massage also release oxytocin in a baby's system to calm him and make him more open to your overtures. No wonder skin contact has proved to be such a time-tested and effective tool to overcoming breastfeeding problems! As a baby enjoys skin-to-skin contact, his blood pressure decreases, his heart rate slows, and he begins to feel more open to this pleasurable, warm contact with his mother. One study even found that skin-to-skin provided pain relief to babies undergoing painful procedures (Gray, Watt, and Blass 2000).

These studies involved full-term, healthy babies, but in studies on more vulnerable premature babies, the effects of skin-to-skin are even more amazing. Research indicates that preemies who spend time in skin-to-skin contact benefit in many ways, including:

- Fewer heartbeat and breathing irregularities (Cattaneo et al. 1998);

- Better oxygen levels and maintenance of body temperature (Törnhage et al. 1999);

- Less reaction to painful procedures (Johnston et al. 2003);

- Lower levels of stress hormones (Feldman et al. 2002);

- Earlier discharge from the hospital and greater likelihood of full breastfeeding at discharge (Charpak et al. 2001);

- A better parent-child relationship (Charpak et al. 2001).

And as we said at the beginning of this chapter, in the developing world, understanding the profound effects of skin-to-skin has decreased mortality rates dramatically in areas where technology is not available. But as we've seen, skin-to-skin isn't important only for premature babies. All human babies are born expecting the calming, comforting habitat of their mother's body, and every baby deserves this loving transition to life outside the womb.

WHEN THE SYSTEM BREAKS DOWN

Most of us don't think much about the role of physical touch in our lives, and its effect is much more profound than you might imagine. Right from birth, skin-to-skin contact encourages a close relationship between mother and baby and promotes breastfeeding, but it is more than a pleasant nice-to-have. Touch is vital to your baby's physical and emotional development. Of course, there are times when a mother and baby cannot be together after birth, and this loss can be made up after they are reunited. But if you have a choice, there are many reasons to do everything possible to keep your baby close from birth.

What are the downsides to the newborn of lack of touch? When full-term, healthy babies are not held, they cry more, are more stressed, and have higher blood pressure. If lack of touch becomes chronic, they are at a greater risk of feeding problems. Premature babies who do not participate in kangaroo care have lower survival rates, more heartbeat and breathing difficulties, more problems with oxygenation, greater stress levels, more pain experienced during procedures, later discharge from the hospital, premature weaning, and relationship problems between parent and child (Cattaneo et al. 1998; Törnhage et al. 1999; Johnston et al. 2003; Feldman et al. 2002; Charpak et al. 2001).

Long-term Effects of Touch

In the last chapter, we described a study of full-term, healthy babies at birth in which a short separation was found to greatly affect the first breastfeeding (Righard and Alade 1990). These practices, which are still all too common, reflect a cultural insensitivity to the importance of touch and togetherness. It seems obvious that mothers and babies cannot breastfeed when they're separated and that being apart could affect breastfeeding. Yet in many hospitals and birthing facilities, little effort is made to keep mothers and babies together. Indeed, giving mother and baby time to touch and to get acquainted after birth sometimes seems more like an afterthought. That is why it is worth your while to make arrangements to stay with your baby as much as possible after birth (even if it's not standard procedure) and to arrange for your support person to act as your advocate as needed.

EFFECTS OF TOUCH ON FEEDING

Although most parents are understandably happy to cuddle with and hold their babies as a normal part of family life, some popular parenting books and programs discourage touching, except at specific, prescribed times. When weighing your parenting options, it may help to know that restricted physical contact can contribute to a variety of problems. Lack of touch has been linked to feeding disorders, refusal to feed, malnutrition, and failure to thrive (Feldman et al. 2004; Polan and Ward 1994). These are not just breastfeeding problems but also include problems with feeding of any kind, including bottlefeeding and the acceptance of solid foods in the older baby.

EFFECTS OF TOUCH ON ATTACHMENT AND BEHAVIOR

Touch has also been found to play a critical role in babies' emotional attachments. Research has found a correlation between healthy relationships and touch. Mothers and babies who have lots of physical contact tend to enjoy good relationships. Healthy dynamics naturally flow from lots of touch. On the other hand, relationship problems are often found in mothers and babies who spend little time touching. In one study, researchers found that togetherness and touch predicted good attachment between mothers and babies. Physical distance and separation correlated with emotional distance and attachment issues (Feldman et al. 1999). So never hesitate to pick up your baby for fear of "spoiling." That's not the way it works.

Infant carrying, even without skin-to-skin contact, has been found to help mothers be more responsive and positive with their babies. In one study, researchers randomly assigned a group of low-income American mothers of newborns to use either soft baby carriers, which provided more contact, or infant seats, which provided less contact (Anisfeld et al. 1990). At two months of age, babies who were carried cried less and were less likely to have a daily period of crying than babies whose mothers used infant seats. At three months, mothers who carried their babies responded more quickly to their babies' cries than mothers in the infant-seat group. At thirteen months of age, infants who were carried were more securely attached to their mothers than babies whose mothers used infant seats. The authors concluded that using a soft baby carrier helps mothers be more responsive to their infants and promotes secure attachment. These findings occurred without skin-to-skin contact, but skin-to-skin can only strengthen these positive effects.

Don't ever worry that all the time spent holding, feeding, and comforting your baby is time wasted. It is central to your baby's healthy emotional development and contributes to your life-long good relationship.

EFFECTS OF TOUCH ON HEALTH

You may be surprised to know that regular touch is also critical to a baby's very survival. In his book *Touching* (1978), anthropologist Ashley Montagu notes, just as Dr. Bergman found in Africa, that even in developed countries, touch—or lack of touch—can make the difference between life and death. Dr. Montagu reports that in the 1930s, a New York hospital decreased its infant mortality rate by providing scheduled carrying and cuddling time to the babies in its pediatric ward. Just by adding some affectionate human touch to its medical care, the hospital's infant mortality rate decreased from 30 percent to less than 10 percent. Dr. Montagu writes:

What the child requires if it is to prosper, it was found, is to be handled, and carried and caressed, and cuddled, and cooed to.... It would seem that even in the absence of a great deal else, these are the reassuringly basic experiences the infant must enjoy if it is to survive in some semblance of health. (p. 79)

So, you see, touch is far more than a nice "extra." It is vital for your baby's normal growth and development. How wonderful that science confirms what your heart is already telling you.

Touch and Your Family

Some of the previous studies and examples reflect extreme circumstances. Of course, we know (thank goodness!) that few mothers and babies will find themselves on the "little touch" to "no-touch" end of the touch spectrum. But it is instructive to know first of all that there *is* a spectrum, and second to know which end is healthy and which end is not. That gives you a chance, as you ponder different parenting styles, to think about where on the touch spectrum you want your family to be. Once you decide, you can make your parenting choices accordingly.

When it comes to touch, research tells us that the societies and individuals on the healthy end of the spectrum are those that keep mothers and babies together and spend lots of time touching. Human biology tells us that the human baby is born expecting human milk and constant contact. That is our biological norm. Although constant togetherness and touching may not be how you were raised or how you're expecting to raise your baby, it may be of interest to know that societies exist in which babies are never separated from their mothers. The mothers most definitely work (and work hard), but rather than leave their babies, they simply tie their babies against their bodies while they work and breastfeed whenever their babies show feeding cues.

Of course, as we know from the vast differences among the cultures of our world, human beings are nothing if not adaptable to change. But as we'll discuss in chapters 5 and 8, our own culture has made some very radical shifts in the way babies are fed and cared for in a very short period of time. The danger is that some of these changes may strain our adaptability to its limits and lead to a whole host of problems for both society and individuals. But more on this later.

We don't often talk about biology in the same breath as parenting. But it is difficult to talk about "natural laws" without also discussing human norms. We realize that this perspective may not necessarily affect your choices. But it never hurts to have a broader view as you stake out your own spot on the touch spectrum. Our goal in providing you with this information is to help you find your own place as close to the healthy end of the spectrum as your circumstances and your inclinations allow.

CHAPTER 3

Latch-On: The Heart of Successful Breastfeeding

Law 3: Better Feel and Flow Happen in the Comfort Zone

Understanding the first two laws explains in large part how the "dance" of breastfeeding is designed to bring mother and baby close, a great example of how the physical affects the emotional. When mothers and babies first learn this dance, it is similar to learning other kinds of dances. The first time you try the movements, they feel awkward. But once they're learned, they become easy and automatic—at times even thrilling. Mothers who grow up watching women breastfeed learn this dance in the most natural way. But for those of us who grew up watching babies bottle-feed, some basic knowledge can be of great help.

WHAT EVERY MOTHER NEEDS TO KNOW ABOUT LATCH-ON

In chapter 1, we described breastfeeding as a right-brained (heart or body knowledge) activity. This is how most physical learning takes place, including things like learning to ride a bike or learning a language. Another example we've used is karate. A man we know named Michael took karate lessons, which involves learning a series of specific movements known as *katas*. He found that reading about these katas and understanding them mentally was not enough to put them into his "body memory," so that he could do them smoothly and automatically. Only by practicing these movements over and over did he learn them fully, in both a left-brained (head knowledge) and right-brained (heart or body knowledge) way.

The same thing is true about learning latch-on. We've often shared Michael's perspective on body memory at our home visits with mothers having breastfeeding problems. As these mothers learned new ways of putting their babies to breast, this concept helped them feel less frustrated as they practiced (awkwardly at first) these new movements. It helped them relax, be patient, and keep working at it until latching on felt fluid and automatic.

With a whole chapter on this subject, it's important to emphasize that good latch-on is not complicated. Although it may take some practice at first, it quickly becomes easy. And knowing you've got it right is a snap. You know you've got it when breastfeeding is comfortable for you and your baby is thriving.

Latch-On Basics

Because good latch-on is so basic to successful breastfeeding, at almost every home visit—no matter what the problem—we spend some time discussing and teaching latch-on basics. Nearly every mother and baby benefits from this. These basics include the following concepts:

- The "comfort zone" is where the nipple should be in the baby's mouth for comfortable and effective breastfeeding.

- How to use baby's hardwiring to achieve this.

To make this easier for you to understand, please go to our Web site (www.BreastfeedingMadeSimple.com). There you'll find some animation created to show you good breastfeeding technique in action. Why? Learning latch-on from a book is a little like trying to learn ballet with a written description and still photographs. Much of the magic is in the movements, and these cannot be conveyed fully on a static page. Please keep in mind that if you're having latch-on problems, there's no substitute for a home visit with a lactation consultant. But we're hoping that seeing good latch-on technique in action may be the next best thing.

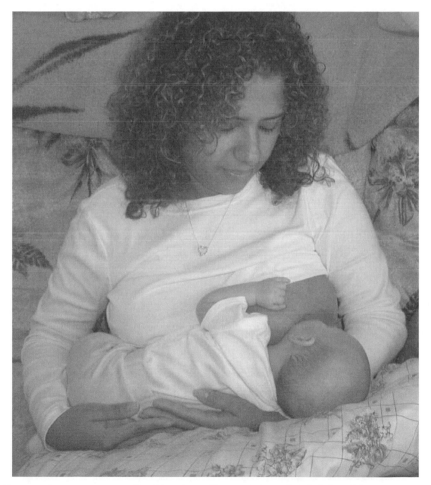

Some mothers are more comfortable using a pillow to support their baby's weight. (©2005 Catherine Watson Genna, BS, IBCLC, used with permission)

THE COMFORT ZONE

The comfort zone is a real place in your baby's mouth. You can find it in your own mouth by running your tongue or your finger along the roof (palate) of your mouth. As you do, you'll notice that the section of your palate nearest your front teeth is ridged or bumpy. Behind these bumps is an area that is smooth. That is your hard palate. As you continue to move back past the smooth area nearer to your throat, you'll notice that the roof of your mouth becomes soft. The comfort zone is near that area in your baby's mouth where her palate turns from hard to soft.

There are two reasons you want your nipple to reach your baby's comfort zone during breastfeeding:

1. It makes breastfeeding comfortable for you by protecting your nipple from friction and compression.

2. It gives your baby more milk, keeping her interested and active at the breast for a longer time.

FINDING A COMFORTABLE BREASTFEEDING POSITION

Before latching your baby on to the breast, think about how you want to hold her. When deciding, keep in mind that some breastfeeding positions may work better than others for you. Because women are born with arms of different lengths and breasts of different sizes and heights, a one-size-fits-all approach is not practical. What works well for your friend or neighbor may not be as comfortable and effective for you.

A hold that works for you. We encourage you to experiment until you find a way to hold your baby during feedings that is comfortable for both you and your baby. In this chapter, we offer many photographs of babies breastfeeding in different positions to give you some ideas. One specific suggestion we make is to find a hold in which your arms and shoulders are relaxed during breastfeeding. Another is to find a position that allows you to hold your baby close to you so that her whole body faces the breast and she doesn't have to turn her head to latch on.

A hold that works for your baby. Touch is the most important sense in triggering a baby's hardwiring. With the right kind of touch, a baby will settle and stay focused. Without it, a baby can quickly become frustrated. The right kind of touch will help baby latch on to the breast in the best way.

Whatever hold you use, your baby's hardwiring will respond best if her head, shoulders, and hips are in a straight line, and her chest and shoulders are pressed firmly against your body. Hold her so that her whole body is facing yours, with her whole body in contact with yours. A baby whose body is turned or twisted is more intent on getting comfortable than on feeding. Firm touch against an uncoordinated newborn's shoulders helps her head, neck, and mouth feel stable, so she can feed better. Enjoy snuggling baby in close under your breasts. The closer your baby's body is to yours, the better.

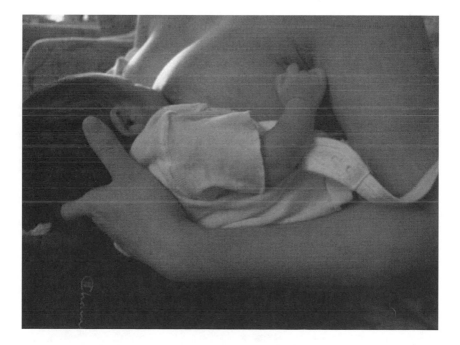

Some women prefer to snuggle their baby against their side for feedings. This works especially well after a cesarean birth and for some women with large breasts. (©2005 Catherine Watson Genna, BS, IBCLC, used with permission)

What to avoid. There are some aspects of your baby's hardwiring that you don't want to trigger during latch-on, as they can work against you. When experimenting with positions, it is wise to avoid the following:

■   Applying pressure to the back of your baby's head

■   Allowing your baby's feet to push against a hard surface

■   Leaving open spaces between you and your baby.

When their heads are pushed, babies tend to push back. There are several reasons for this. For one, pushing on their head tilts it forward, chin to chest, making it more difficult for them to swallow. This may also push their nose into the breast, making breathing difficult. When given the choice between eating and breathing, breathing always wins.

When a baby's feet push against a hard surface, her natural response is to push back, which can work against your efforts to relax and breastfeed. Whichever position you choose, tucking her feet against your body is one way to avoid this.

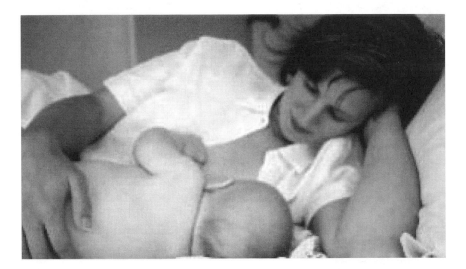

When you learn to breastfeed lying down, you can rest or sleep while you feed your baby. (©2005 Australian Breastfeeding Association, used with permission)

If there are large enough gaps or spaces between you and your baby, she will likely pull up her legs to fill the gap and make herself feel more secure. This pushes her body away from yours, making latching on more difficult.

Your Baby Is Ready to Feed

Whatever hold you choose, the following basic points will help your baby most easily latch on to your breast so that your nipple reaches her comfort zone. As we mentioned earlier, it is ideal to start with a calm, alert baby who is ready to feed. If your baby is upset, use Law 2, "A mother's body is a baby's natural habitat," to calm her first by holding her close and giving her as much skin-to-skin contact as possible. Done? All right, let's start.

To achieve a comfortable, effective latch-on, you'll follow these three steps:

1. Align nose to nipple with your baby's head tilted slightly back.

2. Make sure baby's mouth is wide open.

3. Help baby onto the breast.

ALIGN NOSE TO NIPPLE

Years ago, women were encouraged to center the nipple in the baby's mouth. We know now this is not ideal. Experience has taught us that an off center, or asymmetrical, latch is more comfortable than a centered latch. To achieve this, avoid lining up your baby with her mouth directly opposite the nipple. To find the comfort zone, your baby's lower jaw needs to land as far away from the nipple as possible.

Why is this? Think for a moment about how people's jaws work during feedings. (Take special note of this the next time you have something to eat.) The upper jaw stays motionless; it's the lower jaw that moves up and down. This makes the lower jaw the "working jaw" (Wiessinger 1998). Mothers find that the farther this working jaw is from their nipple when baby latches on, the more comfortable breast-feeding feels. When the lower jaw lands well away from the nipple, it allows the nipple to extend further back into the baby's mouth, to the comfort zone.

Imagine the opposite for a moment. If baby's lower jaw latches on right beneath the nipple, a shallow latch is inevitable. The nipple ends up just inside the baby's mouth, unable to extend back into the comfort zone.

Nose lined up to nipple. What this means, from a practical standpoint, is that when you are lining up your baby's body with yours (in whatever hold you choose), don't align your nipple with your baby's lips. Instead, align your nipple with the baby's nose, or if you prefer, that cute little indentation between her upper lip and the nose known as the "philtrum." When you are lined up this way and the baby's lower jaw drops as she opens wide, you are in perfect position for the best kind of off-center latch.

Head tilted slightly back. Hold your baby so that her head can tilt back slightly. When your baby goes on chin first and head back, it allows you to more easily aim baby's lower jaw where you want it. Why is it helpful for a baby to have her head tilted back? As we described in chapter 1, think about how adults drink, especially when we are thirsty and drink quickly. We tilt our heads back slightly to chug our drink down (try it!), because it is the easiest way to swallow. (On the other hand, try resting your chin on your chest and see how hard it is to swallow.) How you hold your baby can make swallowing easier or harder for her, too. If she is held with her shoulders pressed firmly under your breasts and her hips are pulled in tight against your body, this naturally angles her head out and makes it easier for her head to tilt slightly back.

Chin first. One more thing. If your baby's head is resting on your forearm, a "chin first" approach will probably work better if her head is closer to your wrist than your elbow. If you use a hand to support her head during latch-on, try this with your palm on your baby's back and shoulders and your thumb and fingers behind her ears, or if baby is on her side, with your fingers supporting her lower cheek. As we said before, most babies do not like to have their heads pushed onto the breast and will push back.

To recap the main ideas, when getting ready to latch:

- Hold baby's body under your breasts and firmly against you (shoulders and chest pressed into your body and breast);

- Align baby's nose to nipple;

- Allow baby's head to tilt back slightly;

- Support baby firmly behind the shoulders and back, pull her hips against you, and avoid pushing on baby's head.

A WIDE-OPEN MOUTH

Although most mothers know that babies latch on best with a wide-open mouth and their tongue down, many are unclear about how to make this happen. This is another example of how understanding babies' hardwiring can make a huge difference. Many mothers who are having breastfeeding problems feel as if breastfeeding is out of control. When a mother is unclear on her baby's hardwiring, she may wrongly assume that all she has to do is put the baby near the breast and let nature take its course. But newborns are uncoordinated and usually do better if they get some help from their mothers so that they know what to do. Without this help—especially during the first few weeks—a newborn may respond to a mother's attempts at latch-on by wailing and batting at her breast.

To an inexperienced mother, a baby's frustration at the breast may be a mystery. Some wrongly interpret a hungry, unhappy baby's batting at the breast as a sign that she doesn't want to breastfeed. Usually, nothing could be further from the truth! Some worry that it's her way of saying that she just doesn't like breastfeeding. A mother's worst fear is that it means her baby doesn't like *her*!

Use your baby's hardwiring. The good news is that understanding a baby's hardwiring puts you in the driver's seat. Once you know your baby's triggers, you can make them work for you, eliminating most of the frustration and making latching on easier and calmer for both you and your baby. Learning these strategies can turn an out-of-control mother into a confident, competent breastfeeding woman.

How do you do this? Let's assume first that you have all the right ingredients in place.

- Baby is alert and ready to feed.

- She is held near the breast, with her head, neck, and hips in a straight line and her body pulled in close enough so that there are no gaps between you and her.

- Her head is directly facing the breast, and her body is firmly pressed into yours, with her nose aligned with the nipple.

- Her head is slightly tilted back, and she is approaching the breast chin first.

All you need to do to trigger baby's hardwiring is use tiny movements toward and away from the breast, touching her chin and mouth lightly with the breast. This repeated light touching is baby's cue to open wide and drop her tongue. Mothers are often amazed at how well this works. When a baby gets the right cues, you may see the light dawning in her eyes. Now you are speaking her language!

Lightly bring baby to the breast. Usually, it works best to move the baby slightly toward and away from the breast, *not* the breast toward and away from the baby. Moving the baby instead of the breast gives you more control over the process. It is less confusing this way, too, because you don't have to shift gears—from moving your breast to moving the baby—when baby opens wide. Some suggest lightly rubbing your nipple along your baby's top lip from corner to corner. There's no one right way, so feel free to experiment.

Another tip that may help: moving baby toward and away from the breast with a light and quick touch usually works better than a firmer, slower touch. Some mothers, after rubbing their breasts firmly up and down against their babies' mouths, have eventually given up in frustration. Baby's hardwiring seems to respond much better to a less-is-more approach. The light touch against the baby's mouth and chin works better at triggering a wide-open mouth than a firm mashing of the breast against the baby's mouth.

HELPING BABY ONTO THE BREAST

After aligning your baby well and triggering a wide-open mouth, there is still one vital step left in reaching the comfort zone: helping your baby onto the breast. This help is especially critical during the first few weeks of life.

At birth, babies have limited control over their movements. As they mature and develop, they gain body control gradually from the head down: first head and neck, then arms, and finally legs. By the time they're about four to six weeks old, babies have much more head-and-neck control than they did at birth and can more actively help themselves latch on.

Before around 1980, the connection between latch and breast-feeding comfort was not yet widely understood. Mothers with nipple trauma were usually told, "Just wait four to six weeks. Your nipples will toughen up and the pain will go away." While it has become crystal clear that nipples never do "toughen up" (no matter how long you breastfeed, calluses never form on nipples like they do on a guitar player's fingers), it is indeed true that in most cases nipple pain will subside with time. Even so, a month or more is a very long time to wait when you are in pain at every feeding. As a result, many women stopped breastfeeding. The real reason the pain subsides after a while is because, as babies develop head-and-neck control, they can achieve a better latch all by themselves, without their mother's help. Their newly gained head-and-neck control allows them to pull themselves further onto the breast, which rewards them with more milk more quickly. This better latch resolves their mothers' nipple pain.

We know now that when a mother actively helps her baby farther onto the breast with a gentle push, breastfeeding can be completely comfortable from birth. A baby aligned well at the breast— nose to nipple, head slightly tilted back, chin first—with a wide-open mouth will not reach the comfort zone if that last, gentle shove of the baby's shoulders is missing. Without it, baby ends up with a shallow latch. That gentle push as she latches on is a vital part of moving the nipple into the comfort zone. Another word we sometimes use to describe this to mothers is "oomph."

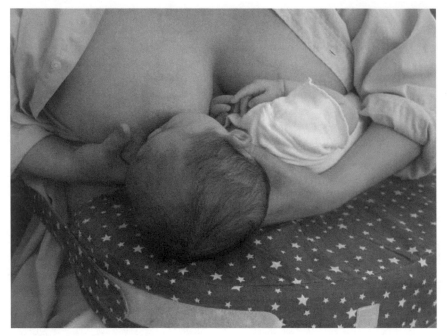

From this angle, the mother has a clear view of her baby's lower jaw. Her palm on the baby's upper back allows her to adjust the "angle" and "oomph" as she helps her baby latch on. (©2005 Catherine Watson Genna, BS, IBCLC, used with permission)

To make latching on easier, remember the three basic concepts:

- Open (a wide-open mouth)

- Angle (nose to nipple, head slightly tilted back, chin first, shoulders and hips pulled in close)

- Oomph (a gentle push on baby's shoulders at latch-on to move the nipple into the comfort zone)

Once the baby is on with a good off-center latch, you can see some of the areola (the dark area around the nipple) above the baby's nose. Despite what many are told, it is not necessary or even desirable to get all of the areola into the baby's mouth. What's most important is that the baby's lower jaw takes in a big mouthful of breast. This is vital to reaching the comfort zone.

Once your baby is on the breast, look to see if her nose is blocked. If so, pull her bottom in closer. This will angle her nose away from the breast. With a great latch-on, your baby's chin will be in the

First, line up your baby's
nose to nipple.
(©2005 Catherine
Watson Genna, BS,
IBCLC, used with
permission)

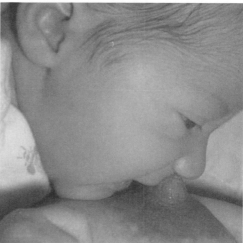

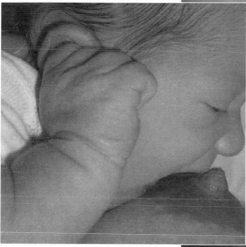

Allow baby's chin to
touch the breast and wait
until she opens *wide*. If
needed, move her toward
and away touching her
chin to the breast.
(©2005 Catherine
Watson Genna, BS,
IBCLC, used with
permission)

When baby's head continues to
tilt back, her upper gum clears
the nipple as she is snuggled in
with a gentle push to help her
draw the nipple into the
comfort zone. Note the dark
area showing above the baby's
upper lip. (©2005 Catherine
Watson Genna, BS, IBCLC,
used with permission)

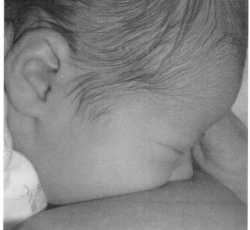

breast, but her nose doesn't have to be. It is perfectly fine to pull your baby's bottom closer to you to give her more breathing room.

Variations on a Theme: Different Ways to Reach the Comfort Zone

While the basics of latch-on never change, different ways to explain them have been helpful to many mothers. We share a couple of these variations on the theme, because one of them may make it easier for you to visualize.

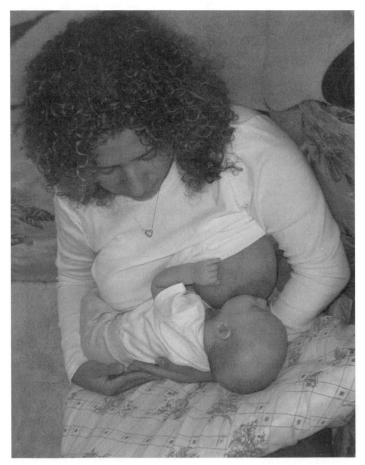

Notice the off-center latch and how the mother pulled in the baby's bottom so that her nose angles away from the breast. (©2005 Catherine Watson Genna, BS, IBCLC, used with permission)

THE SANDWICH ANALOGY

When considering your baby's latch-on, think about how adults take a bite out of a sandwich that's larger than our mouth, suggests Diane Wiessinger, MS, IBCLC, a lactation consultant in upstate New York. What do we do? First, we make sure we are holding the sandwich so that the horizontal plane of the sandwich is lined up with the corners of our mouth. We don't turn the sandwich vertically, because that would make it harder to take a bite out of it. We hold it so that the edges of the sandwich match the corners of our mouth.

Avoid a "wrong-direction sandwich." How does this apply to latching on? If you support your breast with your hand, be sure you are not presenting your baby with a wrong-direction sandwich. If you squeeze your breast, be sure the mouthful of breast the baby is getting is squeezed in the same direction as her mouth. (If your finger or thumb is running parallel to your baby's upper lip, you're good to go.) For example, if you are holding your baby horizontally across your lap, hold your hand under your breast like a U. That way, you will be squeezing the "sandwich" in the same direction as your baby's mouth. Be sure your fingers are out of your baby's way during latch-on.

Get into "sniff position." Think again about how you go about biting into a large sandwich. Like a baby taking the breast, you probably hold the sandwich just above the level of your mouth and tilt your head slightly back. Wiessinger calls this the "sniff position." Also, you don't usually shove the sandwich straight into your mouth. You place as much of the underside of the sandwich you can fit onto your lower jaw and then "roll" the rest into your mouth.

Use a rolling motion. This rolling motion can really help a baby get the biggest mouthful of breast, so that the nipple rolls back to the comfort zone. In fact, in her article on this topic (1998), Wiessinger included photos of her latching on to a water balloon to illustrate (really!). Using lipstick to make a mark on the balloon with her lips, she showed the differences in the end result with both approaches. When Wiessinger pushed the balloon straight into her wide-open mouth, despite her best effort, she took a relatively small amount of the balloon into her mouth. When instead she rolled the underside of the balloon first onto her lower jaw, she drew far more balloon into her mouth, as the lipstick marks showed. In fact, the difference was astounding!

Focus on the underside. The key to reaching the comfort zone is for the baby to get that larger mouthful of breast. One easy way to accomplish this is to roll the underside of the breast into her mouth first, just as we do when we take a bite of a large sandwich. By highlighting an everyday experience, the Sandwich Analogy has helped make breastfeeding more comfortable and effective for many mothers.

THE FLIPPLE

From one of our colleagues in the land Down Under comes another approach to reaching the same goal. Nicknamed by some in the U.S. "the Flipple," it is the brainchild of Rebecca Glover, RM, IBCLC, an Australian midwife and lactation consultant, who demonstrates it in her video *Follow Me Mum* (2002). For order information, see our Resources section.

The Flipple is just another way to get the nipple into baby's comfort zone by rolling the underside of the breast into baby's mouth. But Rebecca adds a new twist. As baby opens wide, the mother presses on her breast just above the nipple with a finger running parallel to the baby's upper lip. This points the nipple up and away from the baby. The mother then presses this finger further into the breast to first roll the underside of the breast into baby's wide-open mouth. Rebecca says in her video, "Don't worry. The nipple is attached. It will follow." Once the breast is in, she uses this finger to help push the nipple inside the baby's upper lip before removing her finger. This ensures that the baby gets a large amount of the underside of the breast before she takes the nipple—a great way to get the nipple into the comfort zone. The Flipple can be especially useful when a mother does not have a very good view of the underside of her breast, but it can be helpful in any breastfeeding position.

THE CHALLENGE OF FLAILING HANDS

For some mothers, babies' flailing hands can present a challenge when latching on. As mentioned before, hungry babies can sometimes be their worst enemies at the breast by batting at and inadvertently pushing the breast away. There are several different strategies you can use if you

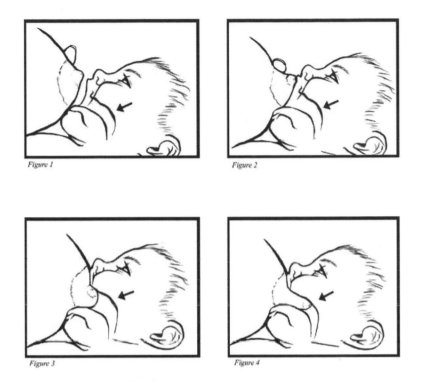

"The Flipple." Arrow indicates the "comfort zone." Before latching, the baby opens wide with nipple above her upper lip. Lower jaw touches the breast first, well away from the nipple (Figure 1). Mother presses her finger into the breast opposite baby's mouth (finger parallel to baby's lips), pointing the nipple away (Figure 2). Using this finger to press into the breast, she rolls the breast into baby's wide-open mouth with the nipple entering last (Figures 3 and 4). Taking a good amount of breast first helps the nipple reach the comfort zone, avoiding friction and compression and promoting comfortable, effective breastfeeding. (©2005 Peter Mohrbacher)

find this to be a problem. Some suggest just giving your baby time to massage and feel the breast, as this is one of your baby's normal breast-seeking behaviors. After given some time to do this, your baby may well move her hands out of the way herself. Catherine Watson Genna, BS, IBCLC, a New York City lactation consultant, offers another tip: If you're holding your baby in front, try sliding the baby's body closer to the opposite breast and snuggling her belly closer. By shifting your baby's body position slightly toward the breast you are not offering, her hands can no longer reach the breast and the process goes more smoothly. If you are holding your baby against your side, pull her further back.

Another way is to use a baby blanket to swaddle your baby and turn her into a "baby burrito." This way, you can keep her hands down and out of trouble. If you use this approach, first undress baby down to her diaper so that she doesn't get overheated during feedings and fall asleep too soon.

WITH PRACTICE, BREASTFEEDING BECOMES AUTOMATIC

After you and your baby have had some time to practice good breastfeeding technique, you'll be amazed at how quickly it becomes automatic. Like karate *katas*, at first you may find yourself very focused on your "moves." But as time passes, you'll find you're concentrating less on what you're doing and more on how rewarding this part of your relationship with your baby is. And before you know it, you'll be one of those mothers who easily fits breastfeeding into their other activities without missing a beat. Breastfeeding will become what it was always meant to be: a normal, natural part of your life with your baby.

WHEN THE SYSTEM BREAKS DOWN

Many of the breastfeeding problems that have become so common are a direct result of shallow latch-on, or the nipple being outside the comfort zone.

If Your Nipple Doesn't Reach the Comfort Zone

A shallow latch-on can cause several issues that can then snowball into other problems.

NIPPLE PAIN AND TRAUMA

With a shallow latch, your baby's tongue will compress your nipple against her hard palate, causing nipple distortion and pain. Nipple distortion is hard to miss. You can see it when your nipple comes out of your baby's mouth oddly shaped, "smashed" looking, or pointed, like a new tube of lipstick. If your baby breastfeeds with a shallow latch feeding after feeding, you may get a "compression stripe" on your nipple, which eventually leads to cracks and bleeding. Other

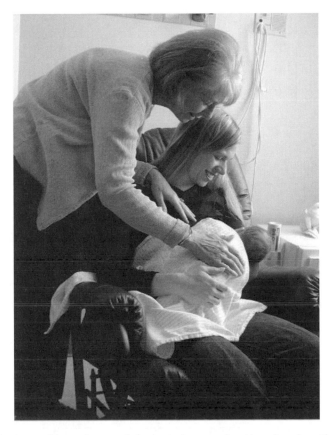

If you're having trouble getting your baby latched on comfortably, a board-certified lactation consultant can help. (©2005 Mary Jane Chase, RNC, MN, CCE, IBCLC, used with permission)

types of trauma can occur, too, sometimes looking like a starburst or scabbing on the nipple. Shallow latch is the most common cause of nipple pain and trauma. If you have nipple pain, please refer to our section on nipple pain in chapter 10 for suggestions on what you can do. If you can't correct the problem on your own within a day or two, it is time to make an appointment to be seen by a lactation professional.

LESS MILK FOR BABY

If your baby breastfeeds with a shallow latch, this may cause pain for you, but it can also be bad for your baby because it usually means less milk at each feeding. When the nipple reaches the comfort zone, it ensures that your baby has a large mouthful of breast. The more breast tissue she has over her tongue, the more milk she can take from the breast. This triggers more active sucking for longer stretches. Taking a small mouthful of breast with a shallow latch-on gives baby less milk when she suckles. There are several consequences of a slow flow of milk during breastfeeding:

- A baby may lose interest quickly, falling asleep at the breast after a few minutes.

- Because the baby is not transferring milk well, she may breastfeed "all the time," taking long feedings with little time in between.

- A baby may gain weight poorly (less than an average of 6 ounces [170 g] per week during the first four months).

SINGLE, DOUBLE, OR TRIPLE WHAMMY

These problems don't always occur together. Sometimes a mother is in pain, but her baby is breastfeeding well and gaining weight fine. Sometimes a mother is comfortable, but her baby is not thriving or is breastfeeding all the time. But sometimes you may wind up with a double or even a triple whammy. It's possible for a mother to suffer from nipple trauma *and* her baby is gaining slowly *and* her baby wants to feed all the time. But whether one or more of these are happening, improving baby's latch-on is the best place to start and the most likely solution.

OTHER COMPLICATIONS

Many of the common problems we'll discuss in chapter 10, from engorgement to newborn jaundice to mastitis to low milk supply, most often have their roots in nipple trauma, poor milk transfer at the breast, or both. The most common cause of nipple pain and trauma and poor transfer of milk is a shallow latch-on. This means that in many cases, these other issues are simply complications of the latch-on. For example, nipple pain and trauma is a significant risk factor for mastitis, because the broken skin on the nipple allows bacteria to enter the breast. Poor transfer of milk at the breast is a risk factor for low milk supply, because your rate of milk production is determined by how full or drained your breast is (see chapter 6).

THE HEART OF SUCCESSFUL BREASTFEEDING

We've devoted so much space to this subject because learning about the comfort zone and how to get your nipple there is the single most important thing you can do for a smooth and easy breastfeeding experience. Even if it takes some time and practice to really feel like a pro, learning the dance of breastfeeding is well worth the effort. Someday your baby will thank you.

CHAPTER 4

The First Week of Breastfeeding

Law 4: More Breastfeeding at First Means More Milk Later

The first few days after your baby is born are a time of tremendous change in your life. At times, you may feel overwhelmed by this huge transition and by all you need to learn. We are here to guide you through this time by giving you some specific information on what is normal and what you can expect. During these first few days, there is one thing that will make all the difference, and that brings us to the fourth law: "More breastfeeding at first means more milk later."

Law 4 is not meant to worry you. You may be concerned that following this law will make your nipples sore. Despite what you may have heard, once your nipple is in your baby's comfort zone, frequent breastfeeding doesn't mean nipple pain. Although mothers were once told to limit breastfeeding in the first days so that they wouldn't become sore, research found that this strategy made no difference (deCarvalho et al. 1984). Without adjusting the latch-on, postponing breastfeeding simply postponed sore nipples. But with your nipple in your baby's comfort zone (see Law 3), you can breastfeed twins and even triplets and not worry about nipple damage. The best way to put breastfeeding firmly on track is to relax, respond to your baby's feeding cues, and feed frequently, which we'll describe in more detail here.

We want to give you a clear picture of what to expect in these first days. (Hint: It probably isn't what you think!) Normal breastfeeding during the first week is different from normal breastfeeding during the second week and beyond. In fact, these differences may feel tremendous. Most of what you have heard or read about normal breastfeeding will be true in your baby's second week. But not just yet.

If your baby is already older than one week while you're reading this chapter, don't skip it. It will probably give you a new perspective on your experience. And if you're having breastfeeding problems, the information in this and the following chapters provides the foundation for overcoming them. We have found that going back to basics is usually the best first step.

To better understand the differences in the first week, let's focus first on the changes your baby faces after birth.

A BABY'S TRANSITION AFTER BIRTH

From your baby's perspective, some startling physical changes happen at birth. Both food and oxygen are no longer constantly provided through the umbilical cord. He begins breathing air with his lungs. And for the first time, your baby begins taking his nourishment by mouth.

Small, Frequent Feedings

During pregnancy, few women question their ability to provide their baby with the right nourishment. After your baby is born, your body is equally well-equipped to give him just what he needs to help ease this major transition. Before birth, your baby never felt hunger. His need for food was constantly satisfied. After birth, your baby feels hunger for the first time. Using his digestive system and intermittent (rather than continuous) feeding are new experiences. To make this transition easier, rather than giving your baby large amounts of milk right after birth, nature starts your baby off gradually, with small, frequent feedings.

SMALL FEEDINGS

For those of us who grew up seeing babies take lots of milk by bottle right from birth, the idea of small feedings in these early days may seem strange, concerning, and to some, even scary. In reality, these small feedings are better for your newborn than larger feedings. Why?

Newborns' tiny stomachs don't stretch. Research on the size of a newborn stomach explains the experience of countless hospital nurses who have learned the hard way: when most newborns are fed one or two ounces by bottle during the first day of life, most of it comes right back up.

During his first day, a newborn's stomach is about the size of a marble. At each feeding he can keep down about one-sixth to one-third of an ounce (5 to 10 ml). Not surprisingly, this is the amount of available colostrum, the early milk, that is ready and waiting for him in the breast.

Not only are newborn stomachs small, but they don't expand like adult stomachs, especially in the first day. In one 2001 study, Samuel Zangen and his colleagues found that during the first days of life, a newborn's stomach doesn't yet stretch the way it will later. The walls of the newborn stomach stay firm, expelling extra milk rather than stretching out to hold it. By three days of age, as the baby takes more and more of these small, frequent feedings, his stomach can expand to about the size of a shooter marble to hold more milk. The following chart gives you a sense of how a baby's feedings increase in amount over the first month.

Baby's age	Average ounces/feeding
3 days	1 oz. (30 ml)
1 week	1.5 oz. (45 ml)
2 weeks	2–2.5 oz. (60–75 ml)
1 month	3–4 oz. (90–120 ml)

Would it be beneficial for you to give your newborn more milk at each feeding and try to stretch out his stomach sooner? No. This is *not* a case of "more is better." Why not? For one thing, small, frequent feedings set up a healthy eating pattern right from the start. Nutritionists now advise adults to eat smaller, more frequent meals, and the same is recommended for babies and children. However, many new parents are encouraged to try to give their babies as much as possible at each feeding and feed fewer times per day. This, however, can lead to overfeeding.

A baby who is encouraged to take more per feeding may be at greater risk for obesity later in life. In fact, research indicates that babies who are bottle-fed nonhuman milks are 25 percent more likely than breastfed babies to be obese by age four to five years (Armstrong and Reilly 2002; Toschke et al. 2002). This may be due in part to the differences between these milks. But it may also be related to differences in feeding method. This tendency to encourage babies to "tank up" to the maximum at each feeding sets up an unhealthy eating pattern at birth that could well contribute to obesity.

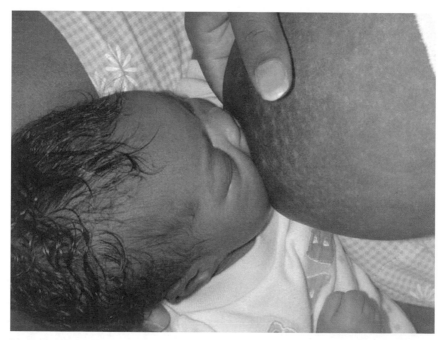

Mother's milk is all babies need during the first days after birth. (©2005 Marilyn Nolt, used with permission)

There are also other reasons small feedings are better for a newborn.

Babies are born waterlogged. Imagine if you had been soaking in a bathtub for nine straight months. That's what life is like in the uterus. Although a fetus is covered with a protective layer of vernix to prevent his skin from becoming white and wrinkled (like ours would be if we spent that much time in the tub), all babies are born waterlogged. The last thing a brand-new baby needs is a lot of fluids. In fact, his first job after birth is to shed some of these extra fluids, which is why most babies lose a little weight in the early days.

Having extra fluid in the tissues at birth is a plus because it allows babies some practice time to learn to get good at taking milk from the breast before their need for fluids is great. Although in many institutions, panic begins to set in if a baby has not fed well at the breast within six to eight hours after birth, it was only about twenty years ago that it was standard practice in U.S. hospitals for newborns to receive nothing by mouth for the first twenty-four hours after birth. The medical professionals at the time knew that fluids were not critical during that first day of life.

This "water weight" babies are born with is the reason newborns (both breastfed and bottle-fed) tend to lose weight during the first three days. This newborn weight loss is considered within the normal range as long as it is no more than 10 percent of birth weight and is confined to the first three to four days of life (DeMarzo, Seacat, and Neifert 1991).

FREQUENT FEEDINGS

One of the most common questions new parents ask is when they should feed their baby. Often they are focused on the clock, because that's where much breastfeeding advice points them. However, breastfeeding has been around a lot longer than clocks, and we're going to describe a simpler way of knowing it's feeding time, one that focuses on your baby. Babies are incredibly smart, and when you tune in to your baby, you'll be amazed at how much he can tell you. Doing this is also a great way to become a more sensitive parent, which will serve you well over your child's lifetime.

Understanding baby's feeding cues. Although many parenting books describe how a new parent eventually learns to tell the difference between a "hungry cry" and a "tired cry," babies should ideally be fed before they are crying at all. In their statement on breastfeeding, the American Academy of Pediatrics (the professional organization that informs pediatricians on what's good practice) states that crying is considered "a late indicator of hunger" and parents are encouraged to feed their babies before they get to this point. Ideally, they say, babies should be fed when they are showing the early feeding cues we described in chapter 1 (AAP 2005).

What are these early feeding cues? Although your newborn cannot talk, when you see these cues, it is your baby's way of telling you he is ready to breastfeed:

- Rooting (turning his head from side to side with a wide-open mouth)

- Putting his hand to his mouth

- Fussing

As we discussed earlier, a baby who is hungry but not yet frantic is going to better respond to his hardwiring and more easily take the breast in the best possible way. In contrast, a baby who is upset and crying has a more difficult time settling down, latching on, and feeding well.

From an adult perspective, less crying means less stress for you. As we discussed, your baby's crying is meant to have a profound emotional effect on you. Nature made us this way so that we would respond promptly to our baby's needs. This is a survival mechanism and it is not healthy to try to override it. Your responsiveness to your baby is an important part of becoming a sensitive parent. This doesn't mean that you need to be constantly on tenterhooks awaiting your baby's cry or that you should beat yourself up if you're unable to catch your baby's cues before he cries. It does mean that training yourself to tune out your baby's crying (his most fundamental way of communicating) increases your emotional distance, which is a less-than-ideal beginning to your relationship.

Less crying also means less stress from a baby's standpoint. There are few people today who believe the old idea that crying is good for baby's lungs. (Some people counter this old chestnut with, "Just like bleeding is good for a baby's veins.") In fact, research has shown that crying is not only stressful for you, it is stressful for your baby, too. Crying raises levels of cortisol, a physical indicator of stress, in a baby's body. So although there will probably be times your baby cries in spite of your best efforts, avoiding crying when possible is good for everyone. The most important emotional lesson of a baby's first year is learning to trust that his needs will be met. And there is no more fundamental need than being fed when hungry.

Rooming in at the hospital. Of course, being able to respond to your baby's feeding cues assumes that you and your baby are together. This may or may not be true depending on where you give birth. For many years, babies were routinely removed to a central nursery at night and during visiting hours. Today, in many places there is more appreciation of mothers' and babies' need to be together to establish breastfeeding. However, it is never wise to assume anything. If you have not yet given birth, it is well worth a phone call to find out what your hospital's "rooming-in" practices are. There are still some institutions in which separation is routine. Even so, it may be possible to make special arrangements so that you and your baby can stay together and have a better start.

Why frequent feedings on the first day are important. One study done in Japan (Yamauchi and Yamanouchi 1990) demonstrated the importance of frequent feedings after birth. The researchers found that more breastfeedings in the first twenty-four hours correlated strongly to less weight loss, more stools, less jaundice, and greater milk intake on days two, three, and five in its 140 babies. We'll describe this study in more detail in the last section of this chapter.

Normal Breastfeeding Patterns

Now let's cut to the chase. What can you expect during these early days? Part of helping your baby transition from the constant feeding in the womb to the intermittent feeding on the outside will involve lots of breastfeeding during these early days. As described earlier, your baby is born with a small stomach. He gets small amounts of colostrum, the early milk, at each feeding. These small amounts digest quickly.

For many babies, this translates to some periods of very frequent and sometimes nonstop breastfeeding.

As we'll discuss in more detail in the next chapter, newborns do not typically breastfeed at regular intervals. While it is true that babies tend to feed eight to twelve times every twenty-four hours, the usual laws of mathematics simply don't apply here. During the first six weeks or so, your baby probably won't feed on any kind of regular schedule. Most new babies tend to bunch their feedings together at certain times and go longer between feedings at other times. If you're lucky, these longer stretches (up to four to five hours is fine) will be at night—but don't get your hopes up at first (see the next section). They'll probably be during the day. So while it is a good idea to keep track of the number of feedings every twenty-four hours (see the later section on this), ignore the intervals between feedings for now. Don't expect any consistency in the intervals between feedings until your baby is older. There may be times of the day or night when your baby breastfeeds every half hour or every hour. That's all just part of normal breastfeeding in the early days and weeks.

If your baby is like most newborns, during these first days there will be times when he is breastfeeding almost constantly, possibly for hours at a stretch, going back and forth from breast to breast. When you try to put him down, he will begin to fuss and show feeding cues. Some people use the word "squirrelly" to describe how babies act during this time. This is not unusual, and if it happens to you, it's *not* a sign that baby isn't getting enough or that breastfeeding is not working. It is a sign that your baby is doing his job well in the days before your milk increases.

Oh, and one more thing. During these first few days, these long feeding stretches are most often at night.

Baby confuses night with day. One recent study confirmed what many new mothers suspect—that most babies are born with their days and nights mixed up. Babies tend to sleep more during the day and breastfeed more at night. In a study designed to help determine what is normal, Australian nurse midwife Stephanie Benson observed the feeding patterns of thirty-seven healthy, exclusively breastfeeding mothers and babies during their first sixty hours after an unmedicated birth. She found the babies fed least often from 3 AM to 9 AM, while their frequency of feeding increased during the day. The babies fed most often from 9 PM to 3 AM (2001).

There are some theories about why babies are born this way. One holds that during pregnancy, babies are lulled to sleep during the day when their mothers are active and moving, and are alert at night, when their mothers lie still. But no one knows for sure why babies mix up night and day. We only know that it is typical for newborns.

Here in the U.S., most mothers arrive home from the hospital on the second day. If this is true for you, this means that during your first night home, your usual sleep time will probably coincide with your baby's peak desire to breastfeed.

Coping with night feedings. What's the best way to handle your baby's feeding frenzy during the wee hours? Most important is your understanding that it's normal and that "this too shall pass." If you have mastered breastfeeding lying down (for more information, including safe sleep strategies, see the next chapter), you're all set. Hopefully, your partner or support person can give you some extra help getting baby latched on well on that first night home so you can sleep and breastfeed without worrying about waking up with sore nipples.

A good strategy is to get into bed at your usual time (or earlier, if you want), arrange yourself and your baby in bed so that it is easiest to pull baby onto the breast whenever needed. Be sure you have whatever pillows you need under your head and behind your back so that you can relax all your muscles and go right back to sleep while baby breastfeeds. (But don't put pillows around your baby, as this could be dangerous.) As your baby wakes you for feedings, put him to breast, or have your partner or support person help you get your baby well latched on. Wedge a rolled-up small towel or baby blanket behind your baby's back (but not his head), so he has the support he needs to stay on the breast. Be sure his head is free to angle back so that he can latch on chin first. He will come off the breast when he's done, and you can hold him against your body and roll over to the other side when he wants the other breast. Or you can lean over toward him to offer the upper breast (see photo on page 110), whichever works best. Most mothers find that it takes some practice to get good at breastfeeding lying down, especially during the early weeks when the baby is most uncoordinated. But it is well worth the effort to learn it, even if you need a second person's help at first (see the next chapter for more specifics, safety tips, and lots of photos). Once you have it mastered, there is no muss, no fuss, and no one has to lose much sleep.

When breastfeeding in bed at night, some mothers worry about how and when to change baby's diapers and what to do about burping. Breastfed babies tend to take in much less air than babies who feed by bottle, so they may or may not need to be burped at all. (With just a little experience, you'll quickly get a sense of your own baby's needs.) During these first few days, a baby is unlikely to be gulping down lots of milk anyway, as it comes in small amounts. So if your baby falls back asleep without burping, let him be. He will wake and fuss if he needs to burp. Regarding diapers, it is practical to have a changing station set up next to your bed. But there is no need to change diapers during your normal sleeping hours unless the baby has a bowel movement. And during these first few days, this is a great job to assign your partner or support person.

Another important way to get the rest you need and to recover from birth is to make a pledge to sleep when baby sleeps. This may be at times when you would normally be awake and getting things done. Keep in mind that you just had a baby and your body and mind will need time to adjust. Be sure to accept all offers of help. This is the time to hunker down and get on your baby's rhythm (for more on this, see the next chapter).

If your baby's internal clock says that midnight to 3 AM is party time, there are some tried-and-true strategies you can use to help baby establish a more amenable schedule. See the next chapter for more on this.

BREASTFEEDING BASICS

Now let's focus on the basics you need to make breastfeeding work.

One Breast or Two?

A common question mothers ask is whether they should give both breasts at each feeding or if they should give just one. The answer is "neither." Ideally, your baby will make this decision. When a baby is healthy and breastfeeding normally, he is fully capable of determining when it's time to switch breasts. After all, he's the only one who knows how much milk he's had and if he's ready to go to the other side.

FINISH THE FIRST BREAST FIRST

Not too long ago, the most common advice given to breastfeeding mothers was to breastfeed for ten to fifteen minutes on the first breast, take the baby off, and then keep him on the other breast for as long as he liked. This strategy worked well for many mothers and babies, but there were some for whom it didn't work.

Disadvantages of breastfeeding by the clock. For the lactation professionals trying to help these mothers, their problem was mysterious. The moms obviously produced a lot of milk, but their babies were not gaining weight well. The babies were also colicky, gassy, and had green, frothy stools. They were not happy campers! Eventually, when the cause of their problem was discovered, we gained a new insight into an aspect of breastfeeding that had not been widely understood.

The issue was that these mothers had been following the standard advice to switch their babies to the second breast after ten to fifteen minutes. Michael Woolridge, Ph.D., a British physiologist, and Chloe Fisher, a British midwife, were the researchers who solved this mystery. In 1988, they described to the world in the medical journal *Lancet* how this way of managing breastfeeding had caused the problem. Fat, they explained, sticks to the milk ducts in the breast. This means that when the breasts are full, the first milk that is released is low fat. As the breast is drained and more milk is pushed toward the nipple, fat is dislodged from the ducts into the milk, increasing its fat content. By switching breasts too soon, these babies had gotten almost exclusively low-fat milk on the first breast. Then they were switched to the other breast, where they also received mostly low-fat milk, having filled their bellies before reaching the higher fat milk. This overload of low-fat milk rushed through their digestive systems, causing the gas, the colic, and the low weight gain.

Babies need the right balance of low-fat milk and cream. Now we understand that the fat content of milk gradually changes during each feeding. When a breast is full, the first milk a baby gets (sometimes called "foremilk") is low fat, like 1 percent milk. As baby continues to feed, the milk increases in fat, changing from 1 percent to 2 percent milk. Keep draining the breast, and the fat content increases until it is as fatty as whole milk, then half-and-half, then cream (sometimes called "hindmilk"). The babies who were having problems received only the low-fat milk. Breastfeeding "by the clock" prevented them getting to the fattier milk on either breast.

Fortunately, once the problem was understood, the solution was simple. The babies were left on the first breast to finish the first breast first. The combination of both the low-fat and the fattier milk no longer rushes through his system. The higher fat content of the fatty milk causes it to linger longer in the intestines, preventing the gas and colic and boosting baby's weight gain.

THE EASY WAY IS TO FOLLOW YOUR BABY'S CUES

In many ways, this finish-the-first-breast-first approach makes breastfeeding blissfully simple. You don't need a clock. You don't need to worry about your milk's fat content. (Later in this chapter, we'll explain in more detail how your baby's stools tell you whether he's had enough of the fatty milk.) Just leave your baby on the first breast until he either pops off on his own and seems finished on that side or falls asleep and comes off. Then change his diaper to see if this extra stimulation makes him interested in taking the other side. (Don't plan to change him right before a feeding, when he's frantic. No doubt by the time he finishes the first breast, it will be good to change him anyway.) If he wakes and is interested in taking the other breast, go ahead and give it. If not, that's fine, too. Once your milk increases on the third or fourth day, most babies take one breast at some feedings and both breasts at others.

This strategy relies on your baby's ability to tell you what he needs. As with us adults, some babies are fast eaters and some are slow eaters. So a clock will never tell you when your baby is done. (How would you feel if, in the middle of your meal, someone pulled your plate away?) Only your baby knows for sure when the flow on one breast has slowed down to the point where he is ready for the other side. Only he knows when he's had the right amount of milk for that feeding. And only your baby knows when he's had just the right mix of the thinner foremilk and the fattier hindmilk. You have no way of knowing, and thankfully, this is one thing you don't need to know. Your baby gets to decide—which is the first step toward healthy eating habits.

Every baby is different. Be suspicious of any parenting books that recommend the same feeding pattern for all mothers and babies, because individual differences can profoundly affect these dynamics. Many mothers with large milk supplies find that their babies always take one breast at a feeding. Mothers with smaller or more average milk supplies often find that their babies always want both breasts. There are no hard and fast rules, because mothers and babies are individuals, and these individual differences are responsible for the natural variations in babies' feeding patterns. (We'll describe this in more detail in chapter 6.)

During these first days, as we discussed, the amount of milk available to your baby tends to be small to match the size of his stomach, and your baby may want both breasts at every feeding. In fact, in these early days, your baby may want both breasts several times at each feeding. Don't hesitate to give each breast more than once if your baby seems to want it. Let your baby be your guide.

HOW TO KNOW WHEN BREASTFEEDING IS GOING WELL

The first time a mother breastfeeds, she often worries about whether it's going normally. For those used to bottles, it may seem unsettling that our breasts don't have markers allowing us to see how much milk goes into baby at each feeding. But fortunately, there are other ways to know that a breastfed baby is getting enough milk. Once you can identify the signs, you can relax and enjoy your baby.

Birth to Day Four

The following sections focus on the areas that are most important and that prompt most women's questions.

YOUR BREASTS

After birth, your breasts will feel soft until the milk increases on the third or fourth day. Sometimes this is incorrectly referred to as the milk "coming in." This description is misleading, because it implies that prior to this, you have no milk. This misunderstanding has led to many newborns being unnecessarily supplemented with formula. The truth is that you have had milk in your breasts during much of your pregnancy. As we described in the introduction, the amount of colostrum, the early milk, your baby receives provides exactly what your baby needs nutritionally and has components needed for the normal functioning of your baby's digestive and immune systems.

During these early days, few women feel much breast fullness. This is helpful for your baby, because it gives him some practice at taking milk from a soft breast before any firmness occurs. With this early practice, your baby will find it easier to handle any changes in breast texture that occur as your milk production increases.

BABY'S WET DIAPERS

You may have heard that new babies should have five or six wet disposable diapers every twenty-four hours and at least three to four yellow stools. *This will be true later but not yet.* Misunderstandings about this are another common reason babies are given formula unnecessarily.

We described earlier in this chapter why, during these first few days, the amount of colostrum, the early milk, is small. He has a small stomach and can't handle more. (It would most likely just come back up anyway due to his newborn stomach's inability to stretch.) He is also born waterlogged and doesn't need more fluids. During this time, he needs to shed fluids to reach a healthier balance.

Because the amount of colostrum baby gets is small at first, the number of wet diapers will also be small until your milk increases on the third or fourth day. Here's what you can expect:

- Day one: One wet diaper

- Day two: Two wet diapers

- Day three: Three wet diapers

- Day four: Four wet diapers

As you can see, as your baby takes his small, frequent feedings, your milk supply gradually increases. By the end of the first week, your baby's output will likely be ten times more in terms of volume than the day he was born.

BABY'S STOOLS

The first stools your baby passes are called *meconium*. These are black, tarry, and sticky and are not made from your milk; they were in your baby's intestines before birth. As you will see later in this chapter ("If Frequent Breastfeeding Doesn't Happen"), passing the meconium quickly is important in preventing exaggerated newborn jaundice. Fortunately, colostrum has a laxative effect, which causes meconium to pass very naturally during normal breastfeeding.

When your baby is breastfeeding well, your baby's stools should begin to change from black to greenish (called "transitional stools") by day three or four. *If a baby is still passing black meconium stools after day four, it's time to take your baby for a weight check. If he has lost more than 10 percent of birth weight, find skilled breastfeeding help to evaluate what needs adjusting (see Resources). Your baby is at risk for underfeeding.* By day five, your baby's stool should turn yellow. In a nutshell, if breastfeeding is going normally, at a minimum, you should see the following:

- Day one: One stool (black)

- Day two: Two stools (black)

- Day three: Three stools (black or greenish)

- Day four: Three to four stools (greenish or yellowish)

If you're keeping track of your baby's stools, which we recommend, keep in mind that in order to count, a baby's stool should be the size of a U.S. quarter or larger (about 2.5 cm). Smaller stools are fine (and your baby will no doubt have stools of different sizes); they just don't count.

If your baby's stool turns to greenish or yellow ahead of schedule, that's great. It just means that breastfeeding is going especially well.

Often new parents are surprised by the appearance of normal breastfed stools. They look nothing like adult stools, and fortunately, they smell nothing like them, either. Rather than being formed, normal breastfed stools are very loose. Some compare them to the consistency of split pea soup, with lots of liquid and some curds. They may look seedy or completely watery. Both are normal. They may also vary in color. Once the meconium is completely passed, normal stools can be anything from tan to yellow to green.

Due to the healthy effect of human milk on a baby's gut, when babies are exclusively breastfed, their stools have a mild, inoffensive scent. Once a baby receives any other food, his gut flora changes, along with the fragrance of his stools.

BABY'S WEIGHT

As we said before, newborns (both breastfed and bottle-fed) typically lose weight during the first few days after birth, while they shed their excess fluids. Researcher Sandra DeMarzo and her colleagues found in one 1991 study that when mothers received good breastfeeding guidance and support, babies lost no more than 7 percent of their birth weight during these first three to four days. A weight loss of up to 10 percent is considered in the normal range, but if your baby has lost 7 to 10 percent of birth weight, it may be time to take a closer look at breastfeeding to make sure baby is feeding well. Some adjustments may be needed.

Babies should reach their low weight by four days of age. *If a baby is still losing weight after four days, seek skilled breastfeeding help immediately.*

If a baby's diaper output is within the normal range, a weight check is not absolutely necessary, although the American Academy of Pediatrics recommends that every newborn be seen by his doctor between three and five days of age (AAP 2005). If a baby has fewer than expected wet diapers and stools, it is worth explaining here that the baby scales available at most baby stores are not accurate enough to rely on during this time. Neither is the strategy that occurs first to many new parents, which is to get on the bathroom scale alone, then with the baby, and subtract the first weight from the second. Ideally, when a baby's weight is checked, a doctor's or lactation consultant's scale should be used and the baby should be naked (no diaper) when weighed. Most scales used by board-certified lactation consultants are accurate to either 0.1 ounce (2 g) or 0.5 ounce (10 g), and doctors often provide free weight checks for their patients.

BABY'S FEEDING PATTERN

Normal feeding patterns can vary in the first few days of life. When breastfeeding is unrestricted, some babies breastfeed for several hours at a stretch, switching back and forth many times from breast to breast, then sleep for several hours, repeating this pattern until the milk increases on day three or four. This is one of the reasons that help is often recommended during this time. Having someone on hand to handle all the other household responsibilities while mother just sleeps and breastfeeds makes this process much easier. Some babies breastfeed for short periods, ten to fifteen minutes, but feed every thirty to forty minutes around the clock. If your baby follows either of these first two common feeding patterns, take heart! This is an intense period, but it doesn't last long. And if you follow your baby's lead and breastfeed like crazy at first, you will most likely be one of the lucky ones whose milk increases quickly and whose baby is soon satisfied for longer stretches. Some babies, particularly those whose mothers received medication during labor or whose labors were very long and difficult, may seem uninterested or sleepy during these early days. However, they need their mother's milk as much as other babies. If your baby is sleeping so much that he doesn't wake for at least eight feedings in twenty-four hours or he falls asleep within the first few minutes of breastfeeding, you may need to help him. Disregard the oft-repeated adage, "Never wake a sleeping baby." In this case, waking a sleeping baby is exactly the right thing to do. See the section called "Sleepy Baby" in chapter 10 for specific techniques to encourage these babies to get the milk they need.

The most important number to track in these early days is the number of feedings. The goal is to make sure a baby breastfeeds well at least eight to twelve times per twenty-four hours.

PASSING LOTS OF GAS IS NORMAL

During these first few days, when a baby is using his digestive system to process food for the first time, it is normal to pass lots of gas. As the baby takes colostrum and its laxative effect begins to work, his digestive system will start to function normally. Gassiness is part of this normal early functioning and is not related to your diet. (See chapter 9 for more on diet and breastfeeding.)

Days Four to Seven

Days four to seven mark the next phase of early breastfeeding. Many aspects of breastfeeding begin to change as your milk increases.

YOUR BREASTS

There is a range of what's normal when milk production increases. When babies breastfeed long and often during the early days, some women never feel particularly full, even after their milk has increased. Knowing this can be a great motivator to follow the natural laws. More typical, though, is some feeling of fullness in the breasts while milk production increases. Mothers usually find during this time that their breasts become larger, heavier, and perhaps tender. Keep in mind that more is happening in the breasts than just making extra milk. Extra blood is also drawn to the breasts to aid in increased milk production, causing some of the swelling you may experience. An I.V. during labor can also cause excess tissue fluid to be retained, causing further swelling.

If breastfeeding does not go well in the early days and the breasts are not well drained of milk, women are at risk for breast engorgement (see chapter 10). If this happens, the breasts become very firm and full. They may also be hard and/or hot. Engorgement can be extremely uncomfortable and is well worth avoiding if possible. If your breasts become engorged, see chapter 10 for suggestions on what you can do. The good news is that if engorgement is treated properly, it usually only lasts for twelve to forty-eight hours.

If a baby is breastfeeding well, normal breast fullness usually only lasts about two to three weeks. Once the hormones of childbirth have settled down and milk production becomes well established, the breasts begin to feel normal and feelings of fullness subside. Some women mistakenly believe that because their breasts no longer feel full that their milk has disappeared. This is definitely not the case. The heaviness and fullness of the early weeks was never meant to be a permanent part of breastfeeding.

BABY'S WET DIAPERS

Once the milk has increased on the third or fourth day, baby's wet diaper count increases dramatically. The baby who had one, two, or three wet diapers per twenty-four-hour day suddenly begins wetting five or six diapers. Several events coincide to make this possible. Your baby's stomach begins to stretch out so that he can take an ounce to an ounce and a half (30 to 45 ml) at feedings, and mother's milk production increases to that level. At one week, the marble-sized stomach of the newborn has stretched to almost the size of a golf ball. More milk made and more milk drunk is reflected in more wet diapers—typically five to six in a twenty-four-hour day.

BABY'S STOOLS

There is also a dramatic change in a baby's stools during this time. In the last section, we described the change in color and amount that occurs from birth to day four. By now, the black meconium that baby was born with should be completely out of his system. The stools of a four-to-seven-day-old baby are made entirely from the milk he has been drinking since birth.

A baby's stools are a very important indicator of his effectiveness at the breast and the state of a mother's milk supply. This is because the stools come from the fatty hindmilk we described in the section "Finish the First Breast First." In order to get to this fattier milk, your baby needs to drink well enough and long enough to drain the breast well. If a baby spends time at the breast but doesn't take the milk effectively (what some lactation consultants call "being at the bar, but not drinking"), he may get the low-fat milk and have plenty of wet diapers, but may never get to the fatty milk. This becomes obvious when the stools don't come or there are fewer of them than expected.

If a baby is not stooling, this is a serious matter. It may mean that he is not breastfeeding effectively. It may mean that his mother is not producing milk normally. Or it may mean both. When a baby is not feeding effectively and draining the breast, most mothers' milk production will not be properly stimulated.

If a newborn five days of age or older has fewer than the minimum three to four breastfed stools the size of a quarter (2.5 cm) or larger in a twenty-four-hour period, it is time to take a closer look. And the first thing to look at is the baby's weight.

BABY'S WEIGHT

A baby's weight is the "acid test" of how breastfeeding is going. How do you know if your baby's lack of stooling is a cause for concern or just an unusual but normal variation? That's easy. You check your baby's weight. A baby should reach his lowest weight on the third or fourth day.

As we said earlier, the American Academy of Pediatrics now suggests that all babies be seen by their health professional within a few days of discharge from the hospital (2005). This makes it possible for problem situations to be caught early enough so that babies are not at risk.

An average weight gain for a fully breastfed baby is about 6 ounces (170 g) per week, starting from the low weight at day three or four. Many breastfed babies gain an ounce (about 28 g) a day or more. A minimal acceptable weight gain is 4 to 5 ounces (113 to 142 g) per week. If your baby is gaining less than that, it is time to seek skilled breastfeeding help.

BABY'S FEEDING PATTERN

You'll probably notice that as your milk increases, not only does your baby's diaper output increase, but you'll probably hear your baby swallowing more during breastfeeding and he will seem content for longer stretches afterward. This is all part and parcel of having more milk. However, as we'll discuss in detail in the next chapter, it is still too early for most babies to fall into a regular feeding pattern. At one week, your baby's stomach is still just a little smaller than the size of a golf ball. (An adult's stomach is the size of a softball!) Because his stomach is small and he is still very immature, it's normal for babies to bunch their feedings together (or *cluster nurse*) during some parts of the day.

One four-to-five-hour sleep stretch is also considered normal, and there is no reason to wake your baby during this longer stretch, as long as he is getting at least eight to twelve feedings per twenty-four hours. This cluster feeding is a normal feeding pattern for most breastfed babies during the first six weeks or so, until a baby's stomach grows larger and with practice they are able to take milk more efficiently. We'll describe this in more detail in chapter 5.

Regarding length of feeding, on average (and not all babies are average) most newborns breastfeed actively (with his jaws moving far enough to make his ears wiggle!) for a total of about twenty to forty minutes at each feeding. Some pauses during feedings are normal. As we discussed earlier, ideally a baby should be allowed to finish the first breast first, get a diaper change (during your normal waking hours) to stimulate interest, and then be offered the other breast. Usually, babies take one breast at some feedings and both breasts at some feedings. If your baby's feeding length is not average, it is easy to tell if this is a normal variation or a cause for concern. Get your baby's weight checked. If your baby is gaining well, then you can stop worrying. When a baby is thriving, all is well.

KEEP A WRITTEN LOG

During the first week or two after birth, while you and your baby are learning to breastfeed, we recommend that you keep track of two things: number of breastfeedings (at least ten minutes total of wide jaw movements) and number of stools at least the size of a U.S. quarter (2.5 cm).

It is actually better to keep this simple, as the more complicated your log, the more difficult it is to interpret. You don't really need to know how many minutes your baby spends on each breast or any of the other small details. A simple log like the following will better help you keep your eye on the bottom line:

1. Get a blank piece of paper of any size.

2. Draw a line down the middle.

3. Decide when you'd like to start your twenty-four-hour day (now is fine).

4.   Mark one column heading as "# breastfeedings."

5.   Mark the other column heading as "# stools."

6.   Make a tally mark for every breastfeeding with at least ten minutes of active suckling (one breast is fine).

7.   Make a tally mark for every stool the size of a quarter (2.5 cm) or larger (start tracking this after your baby's stools have turned yellow, greenish, or tan).

8.   Count your totals at the end of each twenty-four-hour period.

Counting your totals is the most important step. Number of feedings should be eight or more. Number of yellowish stools the size of a quarter or larger should be three to four or more. If your baby is not waking to feed at least eight times or is not feeding long enough, see "Sleepy Baby" in chapter 10 for suggestions. If after day four the number of stools is less than three to four, adjust your latch-on (see chapter 3), use the breast compression technique described in "Sleepy Baby" in chapter 10, and make arrangements with your baby's health-care provider to bring your baby in for a weight check.

After day four, a baby who is having fewer yellow stools but is gaining weight normally is fine, meaning this should be considered a normal variation for this child. *But this state of affairs is rare.*

Note: It is not constipation when the exclusively breastfed baby has too few stools.

Exclusively breastfed newborns do not become constipated. Constipation, or hard, dry stools, is a common digestive side effect of infant formula. Because most health professionals are not trained in breastfeeding norms, many mothers of exclusively breastfed babies are erroneously told when their baby is not stooling that he is constipated and that they should give a suppository. A fully breastfed baby not passing enough stools is a red flag for underfeeding, and his weight should be checked as soon as possible. Giving a suppository only delays getting appropriate help, prolongs the problem, and puts your baby (and breastfeeding) at risk.

COUNT WET DIAPERS?

Some suggest also keeping track of wet diapers, but this is really not necessary. As we explained before, the first milk your baby gets at the breast is the thinner, watery, low-fat milk. The fattier "hindmilk" comes after and it is the fattier milk that creates the stools and puts on weight. So if your baby has enough stools, you know that he has already received plenty of fluids earlier in the feeding.

We like to simplify this way because counting wet diapers can be very difficult, especially when an ultra-absorbent disposable diaper is used. The average amount of urine a newborn voids is only about a tablespoon (15ml). Between the small amount of urine and the absorption of the diaper, it is really hard to tell when one of these diapers is wet.

WHEN THE SYSTEM BREAKS DOWN

The frequent feedings of normal breastfeeding may sound overwhelming, but if your baby breastfeeds well and often in the early days—at least eight to twelve feedings every twenty-four hours—you'll avoid common problems that you definitely don't need.

If Frequent Breastfeeding Doesn't Happen

When breastfeeding is delayed, restricted, unnecessarily supplemented, or baby feeds ineffectively, possible side effects include:

- painful breast engorgement in mother;

- a delay in increased milk production and excessive weight loss in baby;

- exaggerated newborn jaundice.

ENGORGEMENT

When the amount of milk you produce increases dramatically on the third or fourth day after birth, some breast fullness is common. When a mother is engorged, her breasts become very full, very firm, sometimes hard, and sometimes hot. Severe engorgement can also be painful. In the past, engorgement was considered normal for breastfeeding mothers. We know now that it is not.

Mothers often mistakenly believe that engorgement is caused by the increase in milk production. But that is only part of the picture. Engorgement is caused by the congestion of many fluids in the breast, including extra milk, blood, and tissue fluid retention aggravated by I.V.s used during labor. The good news is that engorgement is usually short-lived, provided that a baby is able to latch on and drain milk well from the breast. The more often and well the milk is drained, the more quickly the extra blood and other fluids can drain away, which both prevents and treats engorgement. (For more, see "Engorgement" in chapter 10.)

DELAY IN MILK INCREASE

Lack of frequent feedings in the early days may also delay the onset of more plentiful milk. A study of 140 newborns in Japan shed light on the role of frequent feedings in increasing milk production faster (Yamauchi and Yamanouchi 1990). In this study, when compared with babies who breastfed less than seven times on day one, babies who breastfed between seven and eleven times during their first twenty-four hours took 86 percent more milk on their second day, 54 percent more milk on their third day, and 86 percent more milk on their fifth day. Not surprisingly, the babies who breastfed more than seven times during their first twenty-four hours also lost less weight and regained their birth weight faster.

EXAGGERATED NEWBORN JAUNDICE

If you don't yet know about newborn jaundice, now is a good time to learn. All mammals are jaundiced to some degree after birth. You know a baby is jaundiced by the yellowish tinge to his skin. A little jaundice is normal and is even considered by some to be beneficial. But if the levels get too high, newborn jaundice can be dangerous. High jaundice levels may mean frequent blood tests for your baby, repeated trips to the doctor, rental of expensive equipment, and even rehospitalization—all best avoided. Although it is very rare, babies have even died from the effects of very severe jaundice.

When babies don't breastfeed frequently in the first few days, they are more likely to have exaggerated newborn jaundice. That is because *bilirubin*, the substance responsible for jaundice, builds up without frequent feeding. Excess bilirubin leaves a baby's system via his stools, and colostrum, the early milk, has a laxative effect, thereby speeding this process. The study cited in the previous section (Yamauchi and Yamanouchi 1990) found a strong correlation between fewer breastfeedings in the first twenty-four hours and newborn jaundice on day six. The more a baby breastfeeds, the more stools he passes, and the lower his bilirubin level.

These numbers may help you see this relationship more clearly. In this study, exaggerated jaundice on day six was confirmed in:

- 28 percent of the babies who breastfed zero to two times in the first twenty-four hours;

- 24.5 percent of the babies who breastfed three to four times;

- 15 percent of the babies who breastfed five to six times;

- 12 percent of the babies who breastfed seven to eight times;

- 0 percent of the babies who breastfed nine to eleven times.

In other words, the more times during that first day the babies breastfed, the fewer of them developed exaggerated jaundice on day six. Not surprisingly, more breastfeedings on day one also correlated strongly with the passage of more stools. And the benefits of frequent breastfeeding extend beyond the first day.

If your baby is jaundiced, see our section "Exaggerated Newborn Jaundice" in chapter 10 for more information on what you can do. The American Academy of Pediatrics has published treatment guidelines for newborn jaundice (AAP 2004), but not all doctors know about them. We also have these guidelines on our Web site. Print these out and talk with your baby's doctor about them.

SUMMARY

Frequent breastfeeding during your baby's first days can prevent many of the problems many people assume are the normal consequences of breastfeeding in the early weeks. Knowing what you can expect from your baby and yourself in this first week can let you know when things are going well or when it's time to seek support from a knowledgeable lactation specialist.

CHAPTER 5

How Your Baby Sets Your Milk Supply

Law 5: Every Breastfeeding Couple Has Its Own Rhythm

THE ADJUSTMENT PERIOD

All of us approach breastfeeding with expectations about what it will be like, but reality often proves to be far different. To make it work, you need to find and follow your baby's natural feeding rhythm. What does that mean? That's the main focus of this chapter.

In the last chapter, we discussed how the size of a newborn's stomach affects her feeding pattern during the first week. In this chapter, as we move forward in time, the baby's stomach size is still a major player. Other factors include her ability to take milk faster and the natural ebb and flow of your milk supply over the course of a day.

For most parents, the first forty days are especially challenging. No wonder it's called "the adjustment period." No matter how a baby is fed, most new parents find that caring for a newborn is surprisingly intense and sleep is at a premium. When you're breastfeeding, both you and your baby are practicing this unique dance, and your baby is at her most uncoordinated. As the weeks go by and your baby starts to gain head-and-neck control, she begins to take a more active part in latching on and breastfeeding gets easier and faster. You and your baby begin to settle in to a new "normal" in your lives. During this intense time of constant feedings and diaper changes, keep in mind that after these first forty days usually comes what we like to call "the reward period."

One physician we know has a standard pep talk he gives new parents who are worried that breastfeeding is too much work. He draws a graph of the postpartum period, with weeks along the bottom and amount of work along the side. Then he draws two lines, one representing breastfeeding and one representing bottlefeeding. His breastfeeding line starts higher, and he acknowledges that at first

The "Work" of Breastfeeding

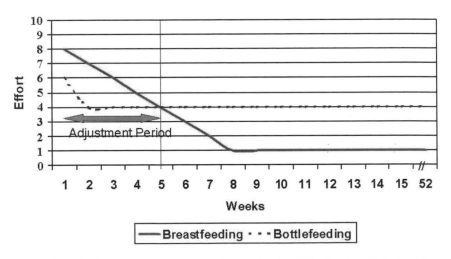

At first, breastfeeding may take more time and effort than bottle-feeding, but within about five weeks—as babies get faster at feedings and need less help—bottlefeeding takes more time. (Concept: Peter Rosi, MD; Graphics: Nancy Wight, MD, IBCLC)

breastfeeding can feel like more work than bottlefeeding. But around five weeks the lines cross. Once mother and baby have become practiced at breastfeeding, it suddenly becomes far less work than bottlefeeding, which requires shopping, preparation, washing, and wide-awake nighttime feedings. After the lines diverge, bottlefeeding stays at the same higher level, while the work of breastfeeding drops.

His main point is that getting breastfeeding established initially is indeed a time investment. But it is an investment that pays back many times over. Breastfeeding saves innumerable hours (and money) over the long run.

During these first forty days, you can make the journey from "adjustment" to "reward" easier or harder, according to the choices you make. These choices most definitely affect breastfeeding, but there is much more to it than that. They also lay the foundation for your relationship with your child. To give you some ideas about strategies that can help, let's see how this time is viewed in other cultures.

The First Forty Days

The first forty days after a baby is born are considered in many parts of the world as a time distinct from everyday life. Mothers are pampered and cared for. They are fed and bathed. They are encouraged to breastfeed and focus primarily on their new relationship with their baby.

Those of us who have had babies in the U.S. are painfully aware of how different it is here, especially the pressure to "get back to normal" as quickly as possible. Within the span of a generation, longer hospital stays and an assumed recuperation period after childbirth have given way to new mothers at the shopping mall right after hospital discharge and women returning to work within their baby's first month. As we will see, this may be one reason why the incidence of "baby blues" and postpartum depression is so high.

Rushing back to what used to be normal is not the best way to handle this vulnerable time. The postpartum period has not always been this way in the U.S., and is handled much differently in other parts of the world.

HOW OTHER CULTURES SEE IT

Is ours not a strange culture that focuses so much attention on childbirth—virtually all of it based on anxiety and fear—and so little on the crucial time after birth, when patterns are established that will affect the individual and the family for decades?

—Suzanne Arms

Many of us in industrialized countries often act as if we have nothing to learn from developing nations. Yet many of these traditional cultures do something extraordinarily right in the way they care for new mothers. After studying postpartum practices in a wide number of cultures, anthropologists Gwen Stern and Larry Kruckman, noted in their classic 1983 cross-cultural review that postpartum depression (including the milder form known as the "baby blues") was almost unheard of in many countries. In contrast, in developed countries like the U.S., 50 to 85 percent of new mothers have the baby blues, and 10 to 20 percent experience the more severe postpartum depression. What makes the difference?

These anthropologists found that all the cultures with a low incidence of baby blues and postpartum depression had several things in common. Not surprisingly, these key factors involved the support and care new mothers receive. Here's what these cultures did to help ease new mothers into motherhood.

The postpartum period is distinct. In almost all the societies studied, the postpartum period is seen as a time distinct or different from normal life. This was also common in colonial America, where it was referred to as the "lying-in" period. This is also a time when experienced mothers help new mothers learn the fine art of mothering.

New mothers rest and are cared for in seclusion. During the postpartum period, new mothers are recognized as especially vulnerable, which is why social seclusion is widely practiced. While they rest, they are expected to restrict their normal activities and stay relatively separate from others, except for midwives and female relatives. Which helps promote frequent breastfeeding. Postpartum is a time for the mother to rest, regain strength, and learn to care for her baby.

Mothers are relieved of household duties. In order for seclusion and mandated rest to be practical, mothers' normal workload must be taken on by someone else. In these cultures, women are provided with someone to take care of older children and take over their household duties. As in the colonial period in the United States, women in other cultures often stay in their parents' homes during this time, where help is more available.

A woman's new status is publicly recognized. In these cultures, much personal attention is given to the mother, which is often described as "mothering the mother." In some places, the new status of the mother is recognized through social rituals, such as bathing, washing of hair, massage, binding of the abdomen, and other types of personal care. The following describes a postpartum ritual performed by the Chagga of Uganda:

> Three months after the birth of her child, the Chagga woman's head is shaved and crowned with a bead tiara, she is robed in an ancient skin garment worked with beads, a staff such as the elders carry is put in her hand, and she emerges from her hut for her first public appearance with her baby. Proceeding slowly towards the market, they are greeted with songs such as are sung to warriors returning from battle. She and her baby have survived the weeks of danger. The child is no longer vulnerable, but a baby who has learned what love means, has smiled its first smiles, and is now ready to learn about the bright, loud world outside. (Dunham 1992, p. 148)

THE REVERSE CINDERELLA

In contrast, the new mother in the U.S. today receives greater concern and support before her baby is born. While a woman is pregnant, people offer to help her carry things, open doors, and ask how she is feeling. Friends give her a baby shower, where she receives emotional support and gifts for her baby. There are prenatal classes and prenatal checkups, and many people questioning her about the details of her daily experience.

Increased focus on the baby. After she has her baby, however, focus on the mother vanishes. A new mother is usually discharged from the hospital twenty-four to forty-eight hours after a vaginal birth, or two to four days after a cesarean birth. She may or may not have anyone to help her at home—chances are no one at the hospital has even asked. Her mate will probably return to work within the week, and she is left alone to make sure she has enough to eat, to teach herself to breastfeed, and to recuperate from birth. The people who gave her attention during her pregnancy are usually no longer there, and the people who do come to visit are often more interested in the baby. There is the unspoken understanding that she is not to bother her medical caregivers unless there is a medical reason.

Is it any wonder that many women find the postpartum period extremely stressful? In one book written for new mothers, *What to Expect the First Year* (2003), authors Arlene Eisenberg, Sandee Hathaway, and Heidi Murkoff describe this transition as "the reverse Cinderella—the pregnant princess has become the postpartum peasant" with a "wave of the obstetrician's wand."

Options for postpartum support. Chances are it will be many years before care will be provided for new mothers through the U.S. healthcare system. But in the meantime, a grassroots movement has arisen to meet the needs of postpartum women. Those who take on this role are called *doulas*, from the Greek word for servant, which is someone who provides practical and emotional help to women before, during, and after birth. A doula can be a friend, family member, or a woman's partner. In some places, professional doula services are available. If you don't have someone to provide hands-on, practical help after birth, and if you can afford it, we strongly recommend hiring a doula. See our Resources section and Web site for ways to find doula services in your area.

We need to learn from other cultures and begin to change the way we think about the kind of care new mothers need. Care should ideally continue throughout the first forty days. The "I-can-tough-it-out" attitude our culture encourages in new mothers will serve neither you nor your baby well. A new mother needs help to recover from childbirth, to make the emotional transition to motherhood, and to breastfeed her baby. Of course, one important task of the postpartum period is learning your baby's breastfeeding rhythm, our next topic.

BREASTFEEDING NORMS

These first forty days are vital to both your adjustment to motherhood and to successful breastfeeding. In this section, we walk you through what you can expect.

Your Milk Supply

In the last chapter, we described how, with frequent feedings, your milk supply increases dramatically during your baby's first week of life. Let's look now at how your baby sets your milk supply during the weeks after.

THE AMAZING FIRST MONTH

The first month is a critical time for your milk supply. After you give birth, your body is primed and ready to make milk. The hormones of pregnancy prepared your breasts by stimulating the growth of your milk-producing glands. When your baby is born, the separation of the placenta from the uterus triggers the hormonal chain of events that causes your milk to increase on the third or fourth day. During this first month your baby's breastfeeding stimulates even more breast growth and development.

The first week. As we discussed in the last chapter, by the end of your baby's first week of frequent breastfeeding, your milk supply will have increased ten-fold—from a total of about one ounce (30 ml) per day on day one to about 10 to 12 ounces (295 to 355 ml) per day by day five.

During this same time, your baby's stomach expands from about the size of a marble to about the size of a golf ball. Your baby can now comfortably take about an ounce to an ounce and a half (30 to 45 ml) of milk at a feeding. As your baby grows, her stomach keeps growing, and so does your milk supply.

The second and third weeks. With frequent feedings, your milk supply continues to build. Now your baby can hold about 2 to 3 ounces at a feeding and takes about 20 to 25 ounces (590 to 740 ml) of milk per day.

This is also a time when babies often increase the number and length of breastfeedings. This is not only because she's hungrier than she was, but also serves to increase your milk supply to meet her growing needs. When this happens, you'll know your baby is doing exactly what she is supposed to do. Experienced mothers have observed that these periods of longer, more frequent feedings (sometimes called "growth spurts") often seem to happen at around two to three weeks, six weeks, and three months.

The fourth week. Your baby is now taking about 3 to 4 ounces per feeding (90 to 120 ml) and her intake has increased to about 25 to 35 ounces (740 to 1035 ml) per day. Amazingly, at around one month you are producing just about as much milk per day as your baby will ever need. (More on this in chapter 6.)

In control of your breastfeeding destiny. There are many good reasons to strongly consider exclusive breastfeeding during the first forty days. In addition to all the health issues, exclusive breastfeeding makes it easier to meet your long-term goals. When your baby sets your supply at "full," you're put in the driver's seat.

With a full milk supply at one month, you can make whatever choices you like in the months ahead. If you want to breastfeed your baby for the recommended minimum of one year, you are set to go. You can always change your mind, but in the meantime, you have everything you need to meet any long-term breastfeeding goal you set.

It may be difficult to increase a set milk supply later. On the other hand, if you find yourself with a partial milk supply at one month, achieving a full milk supply later can be challenging. You are past the point when the hormones of childbirth are working in your favor. Your supply is set. Women who try to bring up their milk supply later find that it usually takes two to three times longer than if they worked on it within the first two weeks. And in some cases, no matter how hard they try, they just can't budge it.

We don't yet completely understand why this is so. There is a theory that during the first week or two after birth, frequent breastfeeding (or pumping) activates a certain number of prolactin receptors in your breast that determine your maximum milk supply for this baby. If a mother does not activate enough prolactin receptors during that time, as the theory goes, she may not establish what it takes to produce a full supply.

Knowing whether you have a full milk supply is easy. If your baby is exclusively breastfed and is gaining weight in the recommended range of at least 4 to 5 ounces (113 to 142 g) per week or more, you're just fine.

THE DAILY EBB AND FLOW

There is more to understanding milk supply than knowing how much milk you make and how much your baby takes every twenty-four hours. A breast is not like a spigot, with the milk at the same level day and night. Your milk supply has its own natural ebb and flow, which affects your baby's feeding pattern.

Morning abundance. Morning is the time when milk supply is usually at its highest. Mothers who express or pump their milk find that they tend to get more milk in the morning than they do later in the day. Mothers who exclusively breastfeed often report that their babies go longer between feedings during the morning hours than in the evening. Why is that?

When scientists have measured the hormonal levels of breastfeeding women, they find that prolactin, the hormone long thought to be related to milk production, is at its highest level in the middle of the night. That may be one factor, but there are no doubt others. As babies turn their days and nights around to be more in tune with the rest of the family, they breastfeed less at night, which means more milk accumulates in a mother's breasts by morning.

Evening low ebb. In the evening, milk supply is at its lowest ebb, and to get the milk they need, babies need to feed more often. Experienced breastfeeding mothers know that the baby who was happily full for hours between feedings in the morning is often the same baby who wants to feed every hour—or even every half hour—during the evening.

Mothers who express their milk also often report that, as day turns to evening, the amount of milk they can pump decreases in amount.

Sometimes called "the witching hour," this feeding frenzy often happens just about the time a mother's thoughts turn to getting dinner on the table. In some cases, these frequent feedings may continue all evening.

The bottom line. What's important about this for your baby is not the ebb and flow; it's the total amount of milk she gets over a twenty-four-hour period. Experienced mothers know how to plan for these predictable evening feeding frenzies. They prepare their evening meal in the morning to avoid the frustration of trying to keep their fussy baby happy while assembling dinner.

For you, the important thing to keep in mind is that "this too shall pass." As you'll see in the next chapter, these evening breastfeeding marathons are usually confined to the adjustment period of the first forty days. Once your baby is bigger, her stomach has grown, and she learns to get more milk more quickly, your breastfeeding rhythm will change, usually becoming much more predictable.

Why a Rhythm vs. a Schedule?

If a mother's breast gave the same amount of milk day and night, and if all mothers produced milk in exactly the same way, a feeding schedule could work well. But that's not reality. This is why—especially while your baby is setting your milk supply—flexibility is important. The ebb and flow of milk supply is one of the natural variations that affect a baby's feeding rhythm. We will discuss the individual differences among mothers in more detail in the next chapter. Suffice it to say now that the amount of milk a mother can comfortably hold in her breasts (which varies considerably among mothers) has a major effect on how often her baby needs to feed to grow and gain weight, as well as to keep up her milk supply. This variation also affects a baby's feeding rhythm.

Because of our culture's focus on getting things done, many new parents feel pressured to quickly get their babies on a feeding schedule. Some strident schedule proponents assert (without any real basis) that schedules, or "parent-directed feedings," somehow promote self-discipline in a child. Some even try to make a connection between feeding schedules and God's design for mankind, even though clocks are a relatively recent man-made invention.

Yet for all the reasons we've discussed, this is the time when a schedule is least appropriate. As British baby expert Penelope Leach writes,

> Over time the behaviors that drive parents crazy change, but they do so when, and only when, the infant's physiology has matured to the point that she is a settled baby rather than a newborn. That may take three weeks or it may take six, but the we-must-do-something approach is likely to prolong the process as well as make it more painful both for parents and infants. (cited in Mohrbacher 1993, p. 41)

As we'll discuss later, there are risks in taking charge and ignoring your baby's natural feeding rhythm.

One major drawback to schedules is that you have no way of knowing at a particular feeding if your baby has gotten the right amount of milk. When your baby is healthy and breastfeeding is going normally, your baby is the only one who knows if she's getting what she needs. When we parents attempt to manipulate this equation, we're in danger of throwing the whole system out of whack.

The concept of feeding schedules is firmly rooted in the "scientific mothering" we describe in chapter 8. To gain a broader perspective on feeding rhythms, a quick biology lesson is in order. With so many ways of raising children, we may wonder if a biological human norm really exists when it comes to infant feeding. But many hints can be found in our biology. So stay tuned and see how we compare to other mammals.

THE IMMATURITY OF THE HUMAN NEWBORN

Some of the differences between us and other mammals are obvious at birth. Human babies are much less mature when they are born than most others. Why? With our larger brains and smaller pelvises, our babies' heads are in danger of growing larger than the mothers' pelvic region can accommodate. The solution? Human babies are born before their brain matures completely and their head gets too big to fit through the pelvis. Most other mammals are born at about 80 percent of adult brain growth. But humans are born at less than 50 percent, with most brain growth occurring after birth. Human babies must finish their gestation outside the womb, and the ingredients unique to human milk play a key role in this.

WHAT KIND OF MAMMAL ARE WE?

To understand this, we again draw from the work of Nils Bergman, an MD from South Africa who has also studied animal biology and behavior (Bergman 2001). Dr. Bergman explains the four distinct ways mammals care for their young. The differences in their milks and in the maturity of their newborns tell us which type of care is right for each. Let's see where the human infant belongs.

Cache mammals. These include the deer and rabbit. Cache mammals are mature at birth. Their mothers hide their young in a safe place and return to them every twelve hours. Consistent with this behavior, the milk of cache animals is high in protein and fat. It sustains the young animals for a long time, because the babies are fed infrequently.

Follow mammals. The giraffe and cow are follow mammals and like others of this group, are also mature at birth and can follow their mothers wherever they go. Since the baby can be near the mother throughout the day and feed often, the milk of the follow mammal is lower in protein and fat than that of a cache mammal.

Nest mammals. These include the dog and cat. Nest mammals are less mature than cache or follow mammals at birth. They need the nest for warmth and remain with other young from the litter. The mother returns to feed her young several times a day. The milk of nest mammals has less protein and fat than cache mammals. But it has more than follow mammals, who feed more frequently.

Carry mammals. This group includes the apes and marsupials, such as the kangaroo. The carry mammals are the most immature at birth, need the warmth of the mother's body, and are carried constantly. Their milk has low levels of fat and protein, and they are fed often around the clock. Humans are most definitely carry mammals. Human milk has the lowest fat and protein content of all mammalian milks. That, and our immaturity at birth, means human infants need to feed often and are meant to be carried and held.

IT'S NOT NICE TO FOOL MOTHER NATURE

As we'll describe in chapter 8, many of our cultural beliefs run directly counter to our biological norms. Human evolution is all about adaptation to change. But in three or four short generations, Western industrialized cultures have attempted to make some very radical changes in how we parent our young. For example, we have made changes over the last three generations from:

- "carry" infant care to "cache" baby care;

- continuous feeding to "nest" care every three or four hours;

- species-specific food to nonhuman milks from "follow" species (cow).

These kinds of radical changes can strain many mothers and babies beyond the limits of their adaptability. Dr. Bergman questions if violating these basic biological norms may have led to the major increases in stress-related illnesses and other problems, ranging from ADHD to child neglect. A growing body of scientific literature indicates that these recently adopted Western parenting styles may not really be such a good idea.

When Breastfeeding Is Going Well

There is no doubt that by breastfeeding your baby, you have taken a significant step in the right direction. And to make the breastfeeding dance most effective and enjoyable, it's important to get into the proper rhythm.

YOUR BREASTS

As we said in the last chapter, if a baby is breastfeeding well, breast fullness between feedings usually lasts only about three to four weeks. Once the hormones of childbirth have settled down and milk production becomes well established, your breasts begin to feel normal and feelings of fullness between feedings subside. At this point, you will only feel full if you have an unusually large milk supply, miss a feeding or two, or go very long between feedings. Some women mistakenly believe that because their breasts no longer feel full between feedings that their milk has disappeared. This is definitely not the case. As we said in the last chapter, the heaviness and fullness of the early weeks was never meant to be a permanent part of breastfeeding.

BABY'S DIAPERS

Just as at the end of the first week, a baby's stools are a very important indicator of how effective she is at the breast and the state of your milk supply. As we explained in the last chapter, the stools are produced from the fatty hindmilk. If a baby spends time at the breast but does not take the milk effectively, she may get the low-fat milk and have plenty of wet diapers but may lack the calories she needs. This quickly becomes obvious when there are fewer stools than expected.

If a baby is not stooling, this is a serious matter. It may mean that she is not breastfeeding effectively, you are not producing enough milk, or both. *If, during the first forty days, your exclusively breastfed baby has fewer than the minimum three to four stools the size of a quarter (2.5 cm) or larger in a twenty-four-hour period, it is time to take a closer look.* And the first thing to look at is the baby's weight.

BABY'S WEIGHT

Just as in the first week, a baby's weight is the "acid test" of how breastfeeding is going. How do you know if your baby's lack of stooling is a cause for concern or just an unusual but normal variation? That's easy. You check your baby's weight. After a baby stops losing weight on the third or fourth day, an average weight gain for a fully breastfed baby is about 6 ounces (170 g) per week. Many breastfed babies gain an ounce (28 g) a day or more. A minimal acceptable weight gain is 4 to 5 ounces (113 to 142 g) per week. If your baby is gaining less than that, it is time to seek skilled breastfeeding help to see what needs adjusting.

YOUR BABY'S UNIQUE BREASTFEEDING RHYTHM

You and your baby are individuals. If babies are allowed to find their natural feeding rhythm, you'll probably find that your neighbor's baby does not feed exactly like your baby, even when both are thriving. The neighbor's baby may breastfeed more times or fewer times. She may feed for a longer or shorter period. You'll also probably notice differences in the feeding rhythms of your first and second babies.

Expect cluster nursing. Because your baby's stomach is still small and she's still learning how to take milk well from the breast, it's normal for babies to bunch their feedings together (or cluster nurse) during some parts of the day. This concept of cluster nursing is the closest thing we've heard to the way most newborns actually breastfeed. As we described earlier, the most common time for babies to cluster their feedings is in the evenings. When she is clustering, your baby may want to feed every hour, every half hour, or even continuously for a time.

Your baby will probably not cluster feed for long. After the first forty days, most babies fall into more regular feeding patterns. Regular, longer stretches between feedings happen as a baby's stomach grows larger and can hold more milk. Feedings also tend to get shorter as a baby gets more practiced at breastfeeding and she can drain the breast faster and more efficiently. Babies outgrow the need to cluster nurse when they can hold more milk and learn to drink more quickly.

Understanding normal feeding patterns is critical, because the most common reason given for giving up on breastfeeding is worries about milk supply. We believe that this is largely due to the general ignorance of normal breastfeeding patterns. New parents are often told that newborns breastfeed eight to twelve times per day (a true statement) and they do the math and assume that their babies will want to breastfeed every two to three hours (not normally true). When their babies begin cluster nursing, parents mistakenly assume that something has gone horribly wrong with breastfeeding. Understanding this law allows you to relax, enjoy your baby, and go with the flow (no pun intended!).

Feeding length and one breast or two. At the beginning of these forty days, on average, newborns tend to breastfeed actively for a total of about twenty to forty minutes. As we discussed in the last chapter, at each feeding ideally a baby should be allowed to finish the first breast first, have their diaper changed to stimulate their interest (during normal waking hours), and then be offered the other breast. Most babies take one breast at some feedings and both breasts at some feedings. As your baby gets older and more practiced, feedings tend to shorten. So the baby who was breastfeeding for thirty minutes may drop to ten to fifteen minutes.

In the normal range vs. average. It bears explaining that while some feeding patterns are "average," there's not necessarily anything wrong if a baby does not follow these patterns. We've met babies who were doing fine who fed faster, fed fewer times, and passed fewer stools. We'll never forget the mother of a three-month-old very chunky baby who, when we asked her how many times per day her baby was breastfeeding answered, "Five." This mother and baby were obviously not average, and yet they were also obviously in the normal range because baby was thriving.

We've also met babies at the other end of the spectrum, who feed longer, feed more, and pass huge numbers of stools and are doing fine. There is a whole spectrum of what's normal for babies, and "average" is just in the middle of the bell curve.

But if your baby is well outside average, don't just assume everything is fine. Have your baby's weight gain checked. (As we said earlier, a bathroom scale is not good enough. You need to take your baby to the doctor's office.) If she is gaining at least 5 ounces a week, you can relax and consider your baby's feeding behavior in the normal range as opposed to average. If your baby is thriving, everything else you're doing is fine.

Normal sleep patterns. One four-to-five hour sleep stretch is considered normal during this time. There is no reason to wake your baby during this longer stretch, as long as she is breastfeeding at least eight to twelve times per twenty-four hours or is gaining well.

Coping Strategies for the First Forty Days

For those of us more familiar with bottle feeding, breastfeeding norms can seem odd and sometimes overwhelming. We offer the following suggestions to help make this adjustment period easier for you and your family.

KNOW WHAT TO EXPECT

Don't underestimate the importance of having good information. Knowing that cluster feeding is normal has saved many breastfeeding relationships. And don't expect a doctor or nurse to necessarily know breastfeeding norms. Most health professionals receive little or no breastfeeding education. This means that it's in your and your baby's best interest for you to learn about breastfeeding. Then, when you are given conflicting advice, you will have a solid basis on which to judge it.

WAYS TO GET YOUR REST

This is not the time to be Superwoman. Make your rest a priority. You're worth it!

Accept all offers of help. Take a page from the book of mothers in traditional cultures and keep the focus on you and your baby by gratefully accepting all help.

Sleep when baby sleeps. In these first forty days, your baby may have her longest sleep stretch during your usual waking hours, and you can take advantage of that to catch up on your rest. Make a pledge right now that you will sleep when your baby sleeps. If your baby is sleeping, stop worrying about writing thank-you notes, shopping, cleaning, or making meals. Get on your baby's rhythm. Remember what other cultures do, and even if no one else around you is doing it, start a new trend by allowing yourself to be pampered.

Adjust your night owl's body clock. If your baby is like most, she was born with her body clock telling her that "night time is the right time."

Once your milk has increased and breastfeeding is going well, you can use some tried-and-true strategies to help her switch from night to day. But count on the fact that it will probably take a few weeks to make a significant change.

The key is to make your usual sleeping hours as boring as possible for your baby. Keep the lights low. To see well enough to latch baby on, use a nightlight or turn on a closet light and crack the door. Keep it quiet. Don't turn on the TV or radio. Change your baby's diaper only when she has passed a stool; wait until morning to change wet diapers. Keep the night hours as unstimulating as you can. Before you know it, your baby will realize that days are where the action is.

BREASTFEEDING LYING DOWN

Of course, all new parents know that their baby will wake in the night to feed. The great news for you is that, unlike the parents who bottle-feed, you don't have to get out of bed to do it. The trick to this is learning to breastfeed lying down. This allows you to sleep and breastfeed at the same time. What a concept! Once you've mastered that, no one will have to sacrifice their rest to feed the baby.

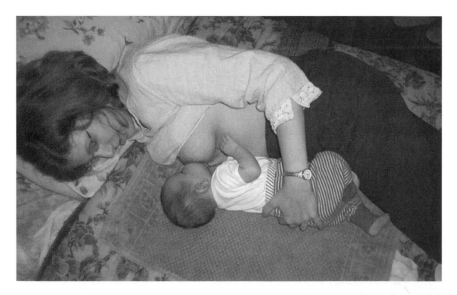

When this mother pulls her baby's bottom in close, their bodies form a V, allowing the baby's nose to angle away from the breast. (©2005 Catherine Watson Genna, BS, IBCLC, used with permission)

A survival skill. Even if it takes you a while to master this, don't give up! Breastfeeding lying down can be one of your best coping strategies for the early months. Once you master it, the issue of when your baby will sleep through the night loses much of its significance. Breastfeeding lying down gets easier as your baby gets older and more coordinated. In the beginning, you will probably need help to get the baby well latched on. But in no time, you'll be able to do this on your own.

Practice when awake. When you are first learning, practice during your normal waking hours. We don't know anyone who learns best when they're half asleep. Once you get settled, you can always take a nap. (You probably need one anyway!) But start at a time when you feel awake and alert.

How-to's. The most important thing to keep in mind is that, like your breastfeeding rhythm, your way of breastfeeding lying down may be unique. How you feel most comfortable will depend on how you're made. Women have breasts of different sizes and shapes, arms of different lengths, and all sorts of body types. So again, be flexible in your approach. Experiment, experiment, experiment! Consider the following description a starting point. Feel free to take it and run with it.

- Start with at least two pillows and a rolled-up hand towel or baby blanket.

- Lie on your side, facing your baby, with a pillow under your head.

- Put the other pillow behind your back.

- Lay your baby completely on her side facing you, and align her body with yours so she is nose to nipple.

- Pull her feet in close to you so your bodies form a V, which may be narrow or wide, depending on your breast size.

- Lean back into the pillow around your back until your nipple lifts off the bed, bringing it to the level of your baby's mouth.

- Put the hand from your upper arm behind your baby's shoulders and rock her gently toward and away from the breast,

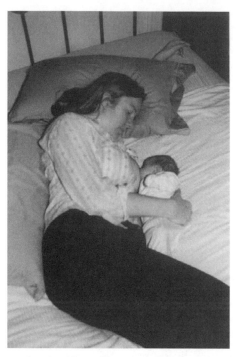

This mother is more relaxed with a pillow tucked behind her back. (©2005 Nancy Mohrbacher, IBCLC, used with permission)

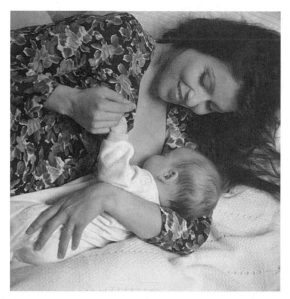

Some mothers feel more comfortable with their lower arm around their baby. (©2005 Medela, Inc., used with permission of Medela, Inc., McHenry, IL)

brushing her mouth and chin lightly with the breast until she opens *wide*.

■ Quickly move her onto the breast by pushing from behind her shoulders to help her get a good, deep latch.

■ Press her shoulders tightly against your body as she latches on.

■ Wedge the rolled-up towel or baby blanket behind her back to keep her in place, leaving her head free to angle back.

There are many different approaches to breastfeeding lying down, as you will see from the photos in this chapter. Try several until you find one you like. The above strategy assumes the baby is lying on the bed, but some mothers prefer to rest their baby's head and body on their arm and use that arm to bring the baby onto the breast (see the bottom photo on page 112). If your baby spits up regularly, you may want to strategically position a bath towel under the two of you that you can easily roll up and replace as needed to avoid having to change sheets.

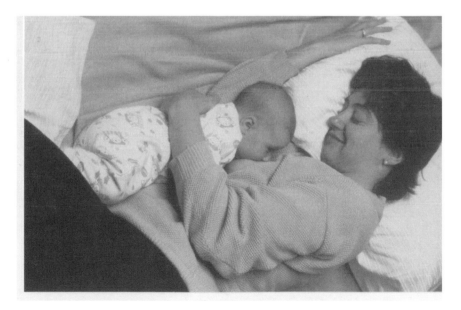

This mother feeds her baby from the upper breast without having to roll over.

There are also other ways. For example, mothers of twins often breastfeed at night resting on pillows propped up behind them, tucking a baby under each arm.

When it's time to switch breasts, you also have choices. You can pull your baby against your body, hold her against you while you roll over, and begin all over again on the other side. Or you can keep her where she is and lean over to feed from the upper breast (see photos on pages 110 and 113). One thing's for sure, breastfeeding lying down is worth practicing until you can do it "in your sleep."

Safe sleep. There are few parents who don't share sleep with their babies and toddlers at least some of the time, even though our culture frowns on it. In some households, bed sharing is reserved for special occasions, illness, or naps. In others, parents and babies sleep together on a regular basis. The idea of mothers and babies sleeping separately is actually a relatively recent one, which again coincided with the rise of "scientific mothering" (which we describe in chapter 8). Mothers don't have to co-sleep with their babies in order to breastfeed, but it does make it easier, meaning mothers lose less sleep and get more rest when they do (Quillin and Glenn 2004). In its 2005 policy statement on breastfeeding, the American Academy of Pediatrics recommends that: "Mothers and babies should sleep in proximity to each other to facilitate breastfeeding."

Just as there are safety standards for cribs and bedding when infants sleep alone, there are also precautions that help ensure safety when mothers and babies sleep together. For more on this, see our Web site for the "Guidelines on Co-Sleeping and Breastfeeding" by the Academy of Breastfeeding Medicine (2003). This organization of physicians lists the following safe sleep recommendations:

- Always position babies on their back or side for sleeping.

- Use a firm, flat surface (avoid waterbeds, daybeds, pillows, and loose bedding).

- Don't fall asleep with your baby on a couch, rocker, or recliner. Your baby could fall out of your ams and become trapped or wedged.

- Limit covers for the baby to a thin blanket (no comforters, quilts, duvets, pillows, or stuffed animals near the baby).

- If the room is cold, dress the baby in a warm sleeper.

- Don't leave a baby alone in an adult bed.

- Be sure there are no spaces between the mattress and headboard or walls, where baby could fall or become trapped.

Also, adults should not share sleep with an infant if they:

- smoke;

- have consumed alcoholic drinks; or

- are on sedatives or any other drug that impairs awareness.

The Academy of Breastfeeding Medicine also suggests some alternative safe co-sleeping arrangements, such as a firm mattress on the floor away from walls or an infant bed that attaches to the side of an adult bed (or co-sleeper). Many families have found safe and creative ways to meet their own need for sleep while also meeting their baby's need to breastfeed. You are only limited by your imagination!

WHEN THE SYSTEM BREAKS DOWN

Cultural forces have a strong influence on how mothers breastfeed and have much to do with the following.

Scheduled Feedings

As mentioned earlier, babies increase a mother's milk supply as needed by breastfeeding more often and for a longer time. If this can't happen due to scheduled feedings, it puts a mother's milk supply and her baby's growth at risk. If a mother's milk supply is low at one month, it may be difficult for her to raise it. With patience, feeding intervals normally become more predictable and lengthen as babies grow and their stomachs can hold more milk (see the following chapter). For the moment, keep in mind that any attempt to put a baby on a schedule is best left until after the first forty days, when a mother's milk supply is set.

Regular Supplements

See the next chapter for more details on how milk supply works, but know for now that whenever your baby receives a supplement, it sends your body the message to make less milk. Milk supply is not about how much fluid you drink or what you eat. It is all about how many times per day your breasts are well drained. When milk is removed, your body responds by producing more milk. If the milk is not removed (because your baby is full from formula or because you are imposing a feeding schedule), your body slows down milk production. The more times per day and the better drained your breasts are, the more milk you produce. That's how women fully breastfeed twins and triplets (and they do!). They just keep putting baby after baby to the breast, and the breast just keeps making more and more milk.

Some mothers breastfeed with a desire to give their baby both breast and bottle. Even if that is your ultimate goal, consider exclusive breastfeeding for these first forty days. Exclusive breastfeeding puts you in the driver's seat. If you discover your baby has a bad reaction to formula (which is true of 7 to 8 percent of babies), you have the option of going back to full breastfeeding until your baby outgrows her reaction to nonhuman milks. The mother who hasn't established a bountiful milk supply at one month and discovers that her baby is allergic to formula is in a very different and potentially difficult situation.

Also, regular bottle use can complicate breastfeeding in the beginning. Even if there is expressed mother's milk in the bottle, during these first forty days while a baby is learning to breastfeed, some babies have a difficult time going back and forth between breast and bottle. This is not true of all babies, and sometimes it can take several bottles before problems develop. Possible problems include breast refusal, ineffective breastfeeding, and suckling changes that cause sore nipples (Righard 1998). Unfortunately, babies aren't born with labels, so you won't know if your baby is susceptible to these kinds of problems until after they occur.

Difficulties are far less likely to happen after the first forty days, once a baby has gotten really practiced at breastfeeding. Despite what you may hear, there is no evidence that waiting to give a bottle until later will make a baby less likely to accept it (Kearney and Cronenwett 1991).

Regular Pacifier Use

Many new parents wonder about using pacifiers. In the same vein, mothers are also frequently cautioned not to let their baby use their breast as a pacifier. We find this odd, and even funny! When we are asked about this, our first thought is, "Which came first, the breast or the pacifier?" Of course the pacifier is a breast substitute, not the other way around.

This begs the question: Can a baby go to the breast to satisfy her urge to suckle without taking milk? There is no question that a baby can drift off to sleep and suckle very softly at the breast so that no milk is flowing. Of course, there is nothing wrong with this. It's comforting and relaxing to a baby. That's why the pacifier was invented—to provide a baby with exactly this experience without the mother being attached.

The pacifier, however, is not a good tool to use during the first forty days. The purpose of the pacifier is to postpone feedings. It masks baby's feeding cues and throws off a baby's unique feeding rhythm. If it is used often enough, a pacifier can reduce the number of feedings per day during the time baby is working to set your milk supply. Once your milk supply is well established, a pacifier is less likely to throw a monkey wrench into breastfeeding. During these first forty days, however, it's best to put away the pacifier.

SUMMARY

Every mother and baby pair is different. Breastfeed frequently in these early weeks to set your milk supply, and allow your baby to help you do this. Beware of any advice that is the same for all mothers and tries to impose a feeding schedule for you and your baby. Many factors, including your own individual milk storage capacity (the topic of chapter 6), can influence how often your baby needs to feed. Just be sensitive to your baby's cues, and let nature take care of the rest.

CHAPTER 6

Meeting Your Long-Term Breastfeeding Goals

> Law 6: More Milk Out Equals More Milk Made

THE REWARD PERIOD

How your body makes milk is one of those basic facts of life that every woman should understand. Yet few do, and misconceptions abound. As we mentioned in the last chapter, the number-one reason women give for weaning their babies earlier than intended is they were worried about milk supply. Researchers found, however, when they compared a group of mothers who were worried that their babies weren't getting enough milk with a group of unworried mothers that both groups of babies were doing well (Hillervik-Lindquist et al. 1991).

This is definitely a case where knowledge is power. Your understanding of milk supply makes it possible for you to make feeding choices consistent with your long-term breastfeeding goals. Part of this understanding includes how individual differences affect milk supply and feeding patterns. Another part is knowing where you fall within the spectrum of normal, so that you can take this into account as you make your choices. This is especially important if you and your baby are not average. One of our goals in this chapter is to share with you some of the new information that strips away the mystery so that you will know how to adjust your milk supply as needed.

But let's begin by describing this new phase in your life with your baby. As you leave the newborn period, breastfeeding becomes much easier—easier, in fact, than bottlefeeding. But there are other issues requiring your attention. With a new baby in your family, your life has changed forever. And as you leave the "mommy zone" of the first forty days and emerge with your baby into the outside world, you and your household must adjust to the new routines that are inevitable when a new member joins your family.

Breastfeeding Is Easier

Around six weeks or so, you and your baby move out of the newborn adjustment period and into the reward period. Feedings are easier, because with practice and growth, the dance of breastfeeding becomes easy and automatic. Your baby has head-and-neck control, so you no longer need to be as careful during latch-on. Your baby is a much more active participant. Mothers who worried about breastfeeding away from home because they needed their special chair or their special pillow now find that they are breastfeeding while walking around the house and that they can easily breastfeed no matter where they are. Breastfeeding lying down becomes a simple matter. A helper and dim lighting are no longer needed for night feedings, because if your baby is laid anywhere near the breast, he latches himself on quickly.

This is the time, as we explained in the last chapter, when breastfeeding becomes easier than the alternative. No one needs to be awake and alert to handle night feedings. There is no mixing, no shopping, no bottle washing, no clogged nipples during feedings, and no worries about running out of formula. (As of this writing, finding formula is a real concern for bottle-feeding mothers in Florida, who are going through their fourth hurricane in six weeks.)

YOUR BREASTFEEDING GOALS

If you have followed your baby's feeding rhythm and allowed him to set your milk supply during those first forty days, you will most likely have a full milk supply as you move into the reward period, which simply means that your baby is gaining weight normally without the use of formula. This puts you in an enviable position. You can decide where you want to go from here. And your possibilities are nearly unlimited. Let's review some of your choices.

If you wean now. You've given your baby six weeks of normal gut function and normal immune-system growth during the most vulnerable time of his life. Keep in mind that, from your baby's perspective, the longer you can delay introducing any formula, the better. Cow's milk (the basis for most infant formulas) is the most common allergen, or allergy trigger, out there for humans. IgA antibodies, one of the many living components of your milk, prevent the absorption of allergens like cow's milk proteins through your baby's gut and into his bloodstream. By restricting these allergens to the gut, they are less likely to pass intact into the bloodstream and trigger an allergic reaction. It takes about six months for a baby's gut to start producing IgA antibodies on its own, which is one reason delaying solid foods until six months is recommended and why research has found that exclusive breastfeeding for the first six months prevents allergies. But even if you stop breastfeeding now, there is no question that six weeks of exclusive breastfeeding is better than none and gives your baby's digestive system some time to mature before being exposed to the allergens of non-human milks.

If you choose to give some formula now. When making feeding choices, also keep in mind that some human milk is always better than none. If you choose to give your baby both your milk and formula, the health risks to your baby of a partial weaning are less than the risks of a complete weaning, as your baby will continue to get some antibodies from your milk. Research has found that at four months of age, babies who are fully formula fed have twice as many ear infections as exclusively breastfed babies. The babies getting both formula and human milk fall in the middle (Duncan et al. 1993).

If you exclusively breastfeed. Your baby's immune system and digestive system will continue to grow and develop normally. The reason the

American Academy of Pediatrics recommends breastfeeding for at least one year (with the addition of solid foods at around six months) is because research has found that for normal immune-system function later in life, we need to receive those living components of human milk for a minimum of twelve months.

However, whether your ultimate breastfeeding goal is six weeks, three months, six months, twelve months, or beyond, to meet your goal you need to understand the physical laws in place and how to use these laws in your favor. And you need to figure out how to make breastfeeding work within the context of your daily life. See chapter 9 for tips for making this easier.

HOW MILK SUPPLY WORKS

As we mentioned in the beginning, there are basic facts of life concerning milk production that every woman should know. Understanding these dynamics gives you both more control over your breastfeeding experience and more satisfaction. When you know how milk supply works, you will spend less time worrying and more time relaxing and enjoying your baby.

There are two main dynamics at work in Law 6, "More milk out equals more milk made." They are how full your breasts are, or *degree of breast fullness,* and how much milk your breasts can comfortably hold, otherwise known as *breast storage capacity.*

Degree of Breast Fullness

Our knowledge about milk production increased dramatically during the 1990s and early 2000s due to the work of a Western Australian research team led by Dr. Peter Hartmann. The Hartmann team, with the help of local breastfeeding volunteers, used a high-tech approach to learn more about how the breast makes milk. In some of their studies they used techniques from the field of topography, which measures mountain terrains, to chart physical changes in the breast and determine how much milk the breasts hold (Cregan and Hartmann 1999). They used ultrasensitive scales to weigh babies before and after feedings to determine exactly how much milk a baby takes at each breast, at each feeding, and over a twenty-four-hour period (Daly et al. 1993). And they used ultrasound to observe internal breast changes during feedings (Ramsay et al. 2004).

Their findings have taught us that one of the primary factors that affects how quickly or slowly milk is made is how full the breasts are, or the degree of breast fullness.

THE FACTORY ANALOGY

To understand more clearly how this concept works, imagine a factory that makes widgets.

Low demand equals slow production. As you enter the factory, you're told that widget sales are slow. You notice stacks of widgets everywhere. Orders for widgets are few and far between, and as you watch, the stacks of widgets grow. With production greater than demand, it's obvious that the workers on the widget assembly line feel no sense of urgency. As the stacks of widgets grow higher, the workers work more and more slowly.

High demand equals faster production. Now imagine that a radical upswing in business occurs. Suddenly widget sales are on the rise. The stacks of widgets in the factory begin to shrink and then vanish. Fewer widgets are available to fill orders, which continue to come in at a faster and faster clip. As demand exceeds production, the workers work faster and faster to keep up with widget sales.

Full breasts make milk slowly. The same thing happens within the breast. As the breast becomes full, production slows down. Why does this happen? Scientists tell us this slow-down is due to a combination of the pressure the milk exerts within the breast and a substance in the milk called *feedback inhibitor of lactation* or FIL for short (Prentice et al. 1989). FIL sends a signal to your breasts to decrease milk production. As the amount of milk in your breasts increases, so does the amount of FIL. The more FIL in your breasts, the stronger the signal to slow milk production. As your breasts get fuller and fuller, like the factory filling with widgets, your rate of milk production slows down.

Drained breasts make milk quickly. The opposite is also true. The Hartmann team found that milk production speeds up when a mother's breasts are drained more fully. If a baby needs to adjust his mother's milk supply, this is how he does it. He feeds more often and he breast-feeds longer, taking a larger percentage of the available milk. As we explained in previous chapters, the milk a baby gets as he drains the breast also increases in fat content. So even if there is just a little milk left in the breast, as he continues to breastfeed, he will get the "high-octane" fatty milk. A little of this fatty milk goes a long way toward leaving baby satisfied. (Think "chocolate éclair"!)

Ever hear someone say, "You need to let your breasts fill up before you feed the baby"? Anyone who says this is seriously confused about how milk production works.

What's average? To better understand the concept of degree of breast fullness, it helps to know what's average. Although many mothers assume that babies take all of their available milk when they breastfeed, the Hartmann team found otherwise. Their research indicates that on average, babies take about 75 percent of the milk in the breasts (Daly and Hartmann 1995). This means that at an average feeding, 25 per-cent of the milk is left in the breasts. If a mother wants to increase her

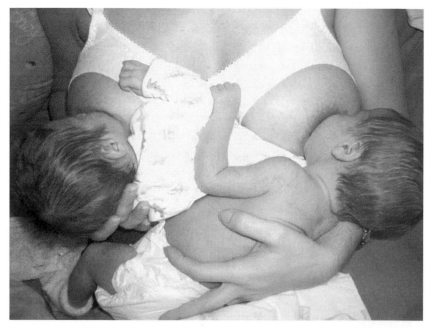

When they know how, mothers can make plenty of milk for twins, triplets, even quadruplets. (©2005 Catherine Watson Genna, BS, IBCLC, used with permission)

rate of milk production, in addition to increasing the number of feedings, she can drain her breasts more fully. This can be done in one of two ways:

- Have baby breastfeed on each breast more than once during each feeding, if he is willing.

- Express milk after the feeding.

The bottom line is: The more drained a mother's breasts are at the end of a feeding and the more times a day they are well drained, the faster her breasts will make milk.

Lopsided? The Hartmann research also tells us clearly that milk supply, while influenced by hormones in the beginning, is most greatly influenced over the long term by milk removal (breastfeeding or pumping). It also confirms that each breast regulates its own supply. In our experience, it is not at all unusual for milk supply to vary between breasts, sometimes considerably. This can happen if, like many mothers, you find breastfeeding on one side more comfortable and tend to favor that side.

You may not realize there is a difference in supply unless you pump or unless the difference is so marked that you look lopsided. But ultimately, it doesn't matter. This is not a permanent change. When your baby weans, your breasts will return to being the same size again. What's most important is that your baby gets enough milk overall, not whether he gets exactly the same amount of milk from each breast.

Breast Storage Capacity

The concept of degree of breast fullness sounds simple enough, but there is also one other recently discovered factor at work that is a major player in your milk production. Have you ever heard that breast size has no bearing on your ability to breastfeed? Well that is true, but the Hartmann team found that the storage space within the milk-making (or glandular) tissue in your breast can affect your baby's feeding patterns. This second factor, called breast storage capacity, goes a long way toward explaining why feeding rhythms vary so much from one mother-baby pair to another.

Breast storage capacity simply refers to the amount of milk you can hold in your breasts. This is not related to breast size, as size is determined more by the amount of fatty tissue in the breasts. This means that smaller-breasted mothers with more room in their glandular tissue can still have a large storage capacity and hold large amounts of milk comfortably. In understanding how breast storage capacity affects your milk supply and your baby's feeding pattern, the key word here is "comfortably."

LARGE STORAGE CAPACITY

A mother with a large storage capacity will likely notice a far different breastfeeding rhythm during months one through six as compared with the mother with a small storage capacity. A mother's breast storage capacity affects feeding patterns in several ways.

One breast or two? First, her storage capacity can affect whether her baby usually takes one breast or two at each feeding. Why is that? Think back to the previous section and the degree of breast fullness dynamic. A full breast makes milk slowly and a drained breast makes milk quickly. Let's say a mother with a large storage capacity can comfortably hold 5 ounces (150 ml) of milk in each breast. Let's also say that a three-month-old baby whose stomach has grown and stretched can now comfortably hold 5 ounces (150 ml) of milk. First, as we mentioned in chapter 4, babies usually take one breast at some feedings and both breasts at some feedings. Many mothers with a large storage capacity report that their babies almost *always* take one breast at a feeding and have no interest in taking the other breast when it's offered. This is because the baby always gets enough milk from one breast to satisfy him.

If a baby always takes only one breast at each feeding, that means there may be long stretches of time before each breast is drained. For example, if the baby takes the right breast at 2 PM and the left breast at 5 PM, there may be six hours or more between drainings. But because a mother with a large storage capacity can comfortably hold more milk, her milk supply will not drop as a result. In fact, spacing out feedings this way will probably prevent the opposite problem—an overly abundant milk supply. If a mother makes far more milk than her baby needs, the baby may have difficulty handling the fast milk flow. Too much milk can also be a challenge to the mother, because she may be more prone to problems such as mastitis (infection of the breast).

Number of feedings per day. A large storage capacity can also have a major effect on the number of feedings per day. As we explained in the last chapter, a baby's total daily milk intake remains remarkably stable from one to six months of age. At around one month, a breastfed baby reaches his peak daily milk intake of about 25 to 35 ounces (740 to 1035 ml) of milk per day, and this stays roughly the same until he begins solid foods at six months and his need for milk decreases as his solids intake increases.

At one month, the average baby's stomach comfortably holds about 4 ounces (120 ml) of milk, so to get enough milk during the course of the day, he needs to breastfeed on average about eight times. (Eight feedings times 4 ounces equals 32 ounces [945 ml] per day.) But as he grows and his stomach grows and stretches, the amount of milk he can handle increases.

A mother with a large storage capacity has more than 4 ounces (120 ml) available at each feeding, and as her baby grows, he may begin to take more milk, say 5 to 6 ounces (150 to 180 ml), at a feeding. If this happens, it will, of course, change his feeding pattern. Since the amount of milk he needs in a day stays the same, if he increases his milk intake at feedings, his number of feedings per day will go down. In other words, the baby who previously needed to breastfeed eight times per day to get 25 to 35 ounces (740 to 1035 ml) per day now needs to feed only six times per day to get about the same amount of milk. (Six feedings times a little more than 5 ounces equals the same 32 ounces [945 ml] per day.)

Obviously, the mother we mentioned in the last chapter whose chunky baby fed five times per day had a very large storage capacity.

Of course, as we described in the last chapter, milk supply ebbs and flows over the course of the day, so a baby will not always take the same amount of milk at every feeding. But hopefully this example clarifies this idea.

Effect on sleeping patterns. Taking more milk per feeding may also affect a baby's need to wake at night to feed. The baby who needs fewer feedings per day tends to sleep through the night at an earlier age than other babies. Yet even with longer stretches between feedings at night, a mother with a large storage capacity may not become uncomfortably full by morning since her breasts comfortably hold more milk. This means she can maintain her milk supply in spite of these longer stretches.

SMALL STORAGE CAPACITY

Now let's look at the other side of the coin. The most important point to remember is that women with a small storage capacity produce plenty of milk for their babies. Researchers noted that none of the women in their studies with a small storage capacity had a problem with low milk supply or slow weight gain in their babies (Daly and Hartmann 1995); their babies were thriving. But these mother-baby pairs had a different feeding rhythm. Let's see what changes.

One breast or two? If the baby of a mother with an average storage capacity takes one breast at some feedings and both breasts at some feedings, what is typical for a mother with a small storage capacity? In general, these babies want both breasts at almost every feeding, especially by one month of age or so, when they can take more milk.

Let's say a mother with a small storage capacity can comfortably hold 2 ounces (60 ml) in each breast. At one month, her baby needs to breastfeed eight or nine times per day to get the 25 to 35 ounces (740 to 1035 ml) per day he needs (two breasts times two ounces times eight feedings equals 32 ounces [945 ml] per day). What is different, however, is that during months one through six, his milk intake per feeding will not change. Unlike the pair in which the mother has a large storage capacity, this mother's breasts hold 2 ounces (60 ml) apiece. So, no matter how big the baby's stomach gets, he will get no more than 4 ounces (120 ml) per feeding.

Number of feedings per day. This individual difference has a profound effect on a baby's daily feeding pattern. To find out how, let's do the math. A baby continues to need 25 to 35 ounces (740 to 1035 ml) per day. He can take a maximum of 4 ounces (120 ml) of milk per feeding. What will happen if his mother attempts to drop some feedings as he grows? (This is sometimes recommended on the premise that older babies don't "need" as many breastfeedings.) Dropping feedings affects this baby in two ways:

1. The baby's overall milk intake per day goes down, because it is impossible for the baby to take more milk at each feeding to make up for the dropped feeding(s).

2. The mother's milk supply decreases.

With fewer feedings, the baby's weight gain will likely slow or stop. Depending on the number of feedings dropped, he may even lose weight. A baby in this situation will be underfed, which means he'll probably also be understandably fussy and unhappy. His sleep may suffer, as well.

The mother with a small storage capacity is also at risk for a decreased milk supply. Why? When a mother drops a feeding, this means the intervals between feedings increase. Remember, full breasts make milk slowly and drained breasts make milk quickly. A mother whose breasts can comfortably hold 2 ounces (60 ml) will feel full very quickly in comparison with the mother whose breasts can comfortably hold 5 ounces (150 ml). If she decides it's time to train her baby to sleep through the night and subsequently goes seven or eight hours between feedings, her breasts will become hard and full after four or five hours. Not only does that put her at risk for mastitis, but her full breasts will make milk slowly. She gives her body the signal to slow down her milk production.

As long as a mother with a small storage capacity continues to feed her baby when the baby shows hunger cues and continues feeding enough times per day, her milk supply will be fine. (The exact number of feedings needed will vary according to storage capacity.) But if she stretches out the time between feedings or drops them to the point that her breasts feel full, her body will respond by producing less milk. She will know she has reached a critical threshold when her baby's weight gain falters.

Effect on sleeping patterns. This is the mother whose baby continues to wake and breastfeed every few hours during the night. Continued night feedings are normal for this mother and baby. The baby needs them to get enough milk and the mother needs them to keep up her milk supply. If this mother has a breastfeeding goal of twelve months, she needs to plan to continue night feedings. (As we explained in the last chapter, many families get creative with strategies for getting their sleep while continuing to breastfeed at night.)

What Is a Full Milk Supply?

Now that you understand some of the most basic dynamics of milk supply, let's discuss a foolproof way to know if you have enough milk: you simply check your baby's weight gain.

NORMAL WEIGHT GAIN

No matter what else is happening with breastfeeding (feeding patterns, sleep patterns, fussy times, etc.), *if are exclusively breastfeeding and your baby is gaining weight normally, you have a full milk supply.*

It also helps to know that normal weight gain has different definitions at different ages. Babies' weight gain slows down as they get older, because their speed of growth also slows down. If a baby continued to gain and grow at his newborn pace throughout his life, he would grow into a giant.

Another point to understand is that our standard growth charts are based on the weight gains of babies on formula, which more current research has found to be slightly different from breastfeeding norms (Butte et al. 2000). The numbers below are based on populations of breastfed babies and they reflect *average* weight gains (not minimally acceptable weight gains). These numbers provide a reliable guide to how breastfeeding is going.

Birth to four days:	loss of up to 7 percent to 10 percent of birth weight
Four days to four months:	6 oz./170 g per week (1½ lbs./ .68 kg per month)
Four to six months:	4 to 5 oz./113–142 g per week (1 lb./.45 kg per month)
Six to twelve months:	2 to 4 oz./57–113 g per week (¾ lb./.34 kg per month)

If your baby's weight gain is less than the above, see chapter 10 for strategies for increasing it.

WEIGHT CHECKS

What should you do if you are worried about whether your baby is getting enough milk? (In our culture, it can be hard not to be worried with all the second-guessing the well-meaning people around us do.) That's simple. Call your baby's health-care provider and make an appointment to have your baby weighed.

Why sit around and worry? Knowing your baby's weight gain will address your concern. If it turns out that your baby is doing well, you can relax and stop worrying. If you find out your baby's weight is of concern, you can seek skilled breastfeeding help right away. If there is a problem, the sooner you make adjustments, the easier it is to get breastfeeding back on track.

YOUR BABY'S DIAPERS

In the last two chapters, we talked about how you can use your baby's stools as an indicator of how breastfeeding is going. As your baby gets older, this is not as reliable. After about six weeks, some babies cut down on their output of stools and yet still do well. If this happens with your baby, it makes sense to get his weight checked to confirm this is normal for your baby. But it is definitely not a cause for panic.

Common Misconceptions

If your exclusively breastfeeding baby's weight is in the normal range, there is no doubt that your milk supply is more than adequate. Remember, at each feeding baby only takes on average about 75 percent of the milk in the breasts. That means there is plenty of milk over and above what your baby is taking. Even so, many mothers worry. What are their worries?

WHY MOTHERS WORRY

These worries about milk supply most often reflect general confusion about normal breastfeeding. Mothers' concerns fall into two main categories: worries about the baby and worries about their breasts.

Baby factors. Because most new mothers today have not had much exposure to normal breastfeeding, they may mistakenly interpret any of the following baby behaviors as signs that they don't have enough milk:

- Baby seems hungry sooner than expected (adjust expectations).

- Baby wants to feed more often and/or longer (normal during a growth spurt).

- Baby suddenly breastfeeds for a shorter time (babies get faster with practice).

- Baby is fussy (almost all babies—no matter how they're fed—have fussy periods).

As we've discussed in the last two chapters, these can all be part of normal breastfeeding.

Some mothers attempt to "test" breastfeeding by giving the baby a bottle after breastfeeding. Their thinking is that if the baby takes milk from the bottle, it proves that their milk supply is low. However, bottle nipples tend to flow fast and many babies will take milk from the bottle even if they had enough from the breast. It is always possible to overfeed a baby with a bottle because of its fast flow.

Another test involves weighing the baby before and after a breastfeeding. Unfortunately, most scales are not accurate enough to detect the small differences between the "before" and "after" weights. Scales available from baby stores fall into this category. As we mentioned before, even less accurate is weighing yourself on the bathroom scale and then holding your baby and subtracting the difference. Scales are available, however, that are accurate enough to measure babies intake at the breast (see our Resources section for information on how to find these). But don't make assumptions about your baby's milk intake at the breast without using the right equipment.

Mother factors. Mothers also worry when they notice the following changes in themselves. However, bear in mind that these are also false alarms:

- Breasts seem softer (this is normal at about three to four weeks).

- Breasts not leaking (some mothers never leak; others stop eventually).

- Don't feel a milk release or letdown (it can happen without your knowing).

- Can't express much milk (this is a learned skill, not a test of milk supply).

Counterproductive strategies. Then there are the strategies recommended to women that are simply wrong-headed and cause unnecessary worry and breastfeeding problems:

- Let your breasts refill before feeding (full breasts make milk slowly).

- One-size-fits-all feeding schedules (differences in breast storage capacities mean one feeding rhythm will not work well for all mothers and babies).

- Measure your milk supply by pumping instead of breastfeeding (milk expression is a learned skill and the Hartmann team found that 10 percent of the women whose babies were doing very well at the breast were unable to pump milk effectively [Mitoulas et al. 2002]).

WHAT EVERYONE THINKS AFFECTS MILK SUPPLY (BUT DOESN'T)

Misconceptions about milk supply abound, even among health professionals. When women ask what they can do to increase their milk supply, the following are usually the first suggestions given:

- Drink more fluids.

- Eat a better diet.

- Get more rest.

Yet except under extreme conditions, these have little to no effect on milk supply.

Drink more fluids. When asked what to do to increase milk supply, chances are this will be the first response, and it seems logical. After all, a breastfeeding mother's body loses slightly less than a liter of fluid a day via her milk. However, research has found no connection between fluid intake and milk supply. In fact, one study found that when mothers force fluids (drink more than they feel inclined to), they had a slight *decrease* in milk supply (Dusdieker et al. 1985). (You read that right!) What is recommended for the breastfeeding mother is simply "drink to thirst." There is no advantage to drinking more.

Eat a better diet. Of course, it's always good to eat a healthy diet. When a mother eats well, she feels better. She has more energy and more resistance to illness. These are good things and should be encouraged. But they aren't the same as increasing her milk supply. A mother's body is made to provide first for her baby. When mothers in developing countries were studied, researchers found that it took famine conditions for three weeks or longer before the quality or quantity of their milk was affected (Prentice et al. 1983). In developed countries, unless a mother is in extreme poverty or has an eating disorder, improving her diet will probably have little or no effect on milk supply.

Get more rest. Just like a nutritious diet, adequate rest is always a plus in terms of a mother's energy and resistance to illness, but there has been no connection found between rest (or lack thereof) and milk supply. Besides, if need be, a tired mother can sleep while she breastfeeds.

You may think that drinking more fluids, improving diet, and getting more rest are harmless enough, even if they don't have the desired effect, but unfortunately, many women assume that if they have tried them, they have done "everything possible." Then, when these efforts don't improve their supply, they end up feeling that their only alternative is to give formula. Another drawback is that mothers may spend a considerable amount of time and effort on improving nutrition and resting that would be better spent improving their breastfeeding technique and increasing number of feedings. Focusing on these things leaves women essentially spinning their wheels in their effort to increase their milk supply.

MEETING YOUR LONG-TERM GOALS

You now have much of the information you need to meet your long-term breastfeeding goals. But there are still a few more points that may help you.

How to Think About Breastfeeding

As you gain confidence in your milk supply and your baby's feeding effectiveness, you will probably become more aware of the emotional aspects of breastfeeding. Once you know that the nutrition part of breastfeeding is covered, you can focus on the closeness and comfort it gives you and your baby. We discussed the amazing impact of skin-to-skin contact in chapter 2 and the relaxing and relationship-building effects of the hormone oxytocin, which is released every time you breastfeed. Research also indicates that breastfeeding mothers are less stressed than bottle-feeding mothers, no doubt in part due to the hormones of breastfeeding and the extra skin-to-skin contact (Heinrichs, Newmann, and Ulridet 2002).

While breastfeeding is a vital source of nutrition for your baby, it is also much more than a feeding method. It's a wonderful way to calm and comfort your baby, to make the transition to sleep easier, and to cement that vital first relationship between mother and baby that sets the tone for your baby's emotional life. In so many ways, breastfeeding is a remarkably effective mothering tool.

NUMBER OF FEEDINGS PER DAY

Some parents worry that allowing a baby to feed whenever he shows an interest might cause overfeeding. One thing we know for sure: a mother cannot "make" a baby breastfeed, which makes worries about overfeeding unnecessary. In fact, as we mentioned in chapter 3, studies indicate that breastfed babies are 25 percent less likely to be obese than their bottle-fed counterparts (Armstrong and Reilly 2002). The properties of human milk no doubt play a part, as well as the baby's ability to self-regulate feedings at the breast, which teaches healthy eating habits. Unlike bottle feeding, a breastfeeding mother cannot see what is left in the breast, so there is no temptation to "tank baby up" to keep him full longer or to avoid waste.

It is also impossible for a mother to breastfeed to meet her own "selfish" needs, an accusation leveled by the uneducated and inexperienced. Yet it is also true that with breastfeeding, there is always more going on than just feeding. Whether a baby wants to breastfeed for thirst (taking only the thin, watery foremilk), hunger (breastfeeding long enough to get to the fatty milk), comfort (to ease feelings of fear or loneliness), or closeness (because he loves you!) is immaterial. Any and all of these needs are legitimately met at the breast and have been for as long as humans have breastfed. You don't need to worry about your baby's reasons when you put him to breast. Breastfeeding is the ultimate in multitasking! As one mother of an older baby said, "I don't count breastfeedings any more than I count kisses." Breastfeeding is a way to give and receive love as well as a way to feed, which is one reason this is called "the reward period." This is when the loving aspect of breastfeeding comes to the forefront.

AMOUNT OF MILK BABIES NEED

As we've explained, research tells us that breastfed babies from one to six months take an average of 25 to 35 ounces (740 to 1035 ml) a day. When this amount was first discovered, it caused concern, because that is significantly less than the amount of formula bottle-fed babies consume.

Human milk vs. formula intake. At age four months, research has found that babies on formula take on average about 33 percent more milk per day than breastfed babies (Neville et al. 1988). This fact has been confirmed many times over, so we know that it's true. This difference in intake is good to know, because sometimes breastfeeding mothers assume they need to pump as much milk for a feeding as their formula-feeding friends' babies take from the bottle. Not so.

Why is this? We are not yet entirely sure. Some research indicates that the metabolism of the breastfed baby runs more efficiently than the baby on formula (Zeskind and Goff 1992). This may mean that formula-fed babies need more calories just to maintain normal function. Because formula is made from nonhuman milks, it may also mean that a baby's system cannot use it as completely, so he needs more of it for adequate nutrition. Future research will clarify the reasons for this difference.

Effect of the delivery system. Another factor that plays a part is the milk delivery system: in other words, whether baby is fed by breast or bottle. We have observed that babies fed human milk by bottle tend to feed with the same pattern as babies who take formula by bottle. They take more at a feeding and feed fewer times per day. In the beginning, breastfed babies tend to average eight to twelve feedings per day, while bottle-fed babies (no matter what's in the bottle) average more like six to eight times per day.

Why is this? As adults, we are advised by experts to eat slowly so that our appetite control mechanism takes effect. What this means is that when you eat slowly, you feel full with less food. Conversely, when eat fast, you tend to overeat, because the signals from your stomach have not caught up with the signals to your brain.

The same thing seems to be true for babies. In general, milk comes faster from the bottle, which has a continuous flow. Babies tend to have more control over milk flow from the breast, which flows faster and slower with milk releases. Dietitians tell adults that the healthiest eating pattern is many small meals over the course of a day. Breastfeeding teaches this healthy eating habit from birth. Bottlefeeding, on the other hand, teaches a baby to overfeed.

For breastfeeding mothers who use bottles regularly, this is important to know. This means you do not need to panic if your baby takes more from a bottle than the amount of milk you can pump at one sitting. If you know that your baby is likely to take more from the bottle than the breast, then you will know that this is not a sign of a low milk supply. If this happens, chalk it up to the difference in the delivery system.

It may be our cultural familiarity with bottles that is at the root of the erroneous advice given to breastfeeding mothers to drop feedings as their babies get older. Just as mothers of an earlier era were motivated to toilet train their babies within the first year to lighten their laundry loads, eliminating feedings by tanking babies up on the bottle helps to eliminate some of the housekeeping work of bottlefeeding. However, with no bottles to wash and no formula to prepare, this is not an issue for a breastfeeding mother.

Starting Solid Foods

We will discuss solid foods in more detail in the next chapter, but know for now that the old recommendation of starting solid foods at four to six months has been revised. The World Health Organization convened a panel of experts to examine all the available research on the ideal age for starting solids, and in 2001 they published their conclusion: delaying solids until six months results in better health outcomes for both mothers and babies (WHO 2001). Research revealed that breastfeeding babies who delayed solid foods until six months:

- had better neuromotor development, and

- had less infectious disease, especially diarrhea.

Mothers who exclusively breastfeed for a full six months:

- had a longer delay in their return to fertility, and

- had a faster weight loss.

When you begin giving solid foods can also affect your ability to meet your long-term breastfeeding goals, because solid foods take the place of milk in your baby's diet. When solids are given too early, you replace a more age-appropriate food with a food that will fill your baby up but that he cannot yet fully digest. The earlier solids are started, the higher the risks of allergies and reduced milk supply, which may undermine your long-term goals.

MYTH: Giving a baby formula before bedtime will make him sleep better, because formula is harder to digest.

FACT: Babies fed by bottle tend to overfeed due to the fast flow, no matter what's in the bottle. Giving a bottle of expressed mother's milk before bedtime would have the same effect without formula's negative health outcomes. If you plan to give formula, wait as long as possible, giving your baby's digestive system more time to mature.

WHEN THE SYSTEM BREAKS DOWN

The following are common choices that often unknowingly undermine women's long-term breastfeeding goals.

Scheduled or Dropped Feedings

The earlier section "Breast Storage Capacity" explains why scheduled or dropped feedings decrease milk supply and thwart some mothers' efforts to meet their breastfeeding goals. Let's look at what happened to one mother in this situation to see how this happens (all too commonly) in real life.

Gabrielle called a lactation consultant because she was in a quandary. She had been breastfeeding her son Ben for six months, but had been struggling with her milk supply since he was three months old. Ben was a sleepy baby from the start and had slept long ten-to-twelve-hour stretches at night. At first he breastfed eight to ten times per day, and Gabrielle knew this was normal for a newborn.

But everywhere Gabrielle turned, she heard or read that she should cut back on feedings as Ben got older. So when she started work at two months, she began to cut back. Almost immediately her milk supply dropped. The first thing she did was to get up in the night to pump her milk, because she didn't want to wake her sleeping baby. For a month she gave him this extra milk and was able to continue to exclusively breastfeed. But as she continued to drop feedings, she also dropped the nightly pumping. By four months, Ben was breastfeeding five times per day and needing more milk than she could pump at work, so she began giving him formula as well.

Gabrielle tried some of the milk-increasing tricks she had heard about, for a while taking fenugreek capsules and later getting her doctor to prescribe metoclopramide, a drug that increases milk production. Every time she used one of these tricks, her milk supply would increase and she would go back to exclusive breastfeeding, but once she stopped, her supply went down again.

The lactation consultant explained degree of breast fullness and milk storage capacity, and Gabrielle realized that she had a small storage capacity. She also understood now what was going wrong. Her strategy of dropping feedings as Ben grew older was working against her. She had a breastfeeding goal of one year, and she still wanted to achieve it. What did she decide to do? She increased her number of breastfeedings at home and pumpings at work and started getting up at night to pump again. (She could have awakened Ben for the night feeding, but she decided she'd rather let him sleep.) Meeting her breastfeeding goal was important to her, and now that she knew how to reach it, she adjusted her routine to make it happen.

Too Much Solid Food Too Soon

In some cases, solid foods started too early and too enthusiastically have drastically reduced mothers' milk supplies and short-circuited their long-term breastfeeding goals. See chapter 7 for strategies to help your baby transition to solid foods in the best possible way and at the best possible time.

SUMMARY

Once a full milk supply is established, the number of times per day a mother needs to drain her breasts and maintain a milk supply can vary greatly, depending on individual differences. New research on breast storage capacity has been able to answer questions about why babies have such different feeding patterns. It also gives us some explanation for why babies differ on when they start sleeping through the night, and why imposing feeding schedules can be a very bad idea for some mothers and babies.

CHAPTER 7

Weaning Comfortably and Happily

Law 7: Children Wean Naturally

Weaning is one of the few experiences that all breastfeeding mothers share. It begins when your baby takes food or drink other than your milk and ends with the last breastfeeding. Although you may think of weaning as an event, it is actually a process. Weaning may be your choice, your child's choice, or it may be mutual. It may be abrupt or gradual, taking days, weeks, months, or even years.

A WEANING OVERVIEW

The word "wean" is derived from a word meaning "satisfaction" or "fulfillment." During most of history, weaning was considered a natural stage of growth, a sign that a child had finally had her fill and was ready to move away from her mother and into the wider world. King David described the sense of fulfillment and inner peace a child gains when weaning comes in its own time when he wrote in Psalm 131:2: "Surely I have stilled and quieted my soul; Like a weaned child with his mother, Like a weaned child is my soul within me."

In the U.S. today, however, weaning is not seen as a process to be celebrated or a naturally occurring stage of growth. Weaning is commonly considered a time of deprivation and unhappiness. It is the approach to weaning, however, that makes the difference. A rigid and abrupt approach makes weaning painful and difficult. But this does not have to be. There are ways to wean that are as gentle and loving as the way breastfeeding began. Weaning gradually—with consideration for the feelings and preferences of both mother and child—can make it the positive experience we'd all like it to be. And that's what this chapter is all about.

When to Wean

Every family makes its own decision about when to wean. This is as it should be, because every family is unique and has its own considerations. As you weigh the relevant factors for you and your family, it may help you to know what the experts say about age of weaning and why.

WHAT THE EXPERTS SAY

Breastfeeding should be continued for at least the first year of life and beyond for as long as mutually desired by mother and child.
—American Academy of Pediatrics (2005)

Why is breastfeeding recommended "for at least the first year of life" by the group that advises pediatricians on good practice? After reviewing the research, its expert panel found that the lifelong health of the child hangs in the balance. Studies indicate that the living properties of human milk are needed for at least one year for there to be a measurable effect on the incidence of immune-related illnesses later in life such as Crohn's disease, Hodgkin's disease, leukemia, ulcerative colitis, and others (AAP 2005). The long-term health outcomes of babies weaned younger than one year were measurably worse. The research that they cited in support of this recommendation was a study of a group of American mothers who ignored cultural norms, and whose babies weaned on average from two and a half to three years of age (Sugarman and Kendall-Tackett 1995).

> ... [E]xclusive breastfeeding for 6 months is the optimal way of feeding infants. Thereafter infants should receive complementary foods with continued breastfeeding up to 2 years of age or beyond.
> —World Health Organization (2001)

Another research-based recommendation comes from the World Health Organization (WHO), whose role is to provide international public-health guidelines. WHO serves developed nations, such as the U.S., as well as developing countries, where in many areas the risks of illness and death are higher due to sanitation problems, fluctuating food and water supplies, and lack of available health care.

WHO's recommendation of "two years and beyond" is based on research into health outcomes of children in developing countries older than one year (Goldman 1983). These studies found that weaned children older than one are at greater risk for illness and death.

- Weaned children between sixteen and thirty-six months of age have more types of illnesses of longer duration and need more medical care than breastfeeding children the same age (Gulick 1986).

- Weaned children twelve to thirty-six months old were three-and-a-half times more likely to die than those still breastfeeding (Molbak et al. 1994).

There is no doubt that the living antibodies in human milk work their magic as long as your child receives your milk. This is important for a toddler, because even with the help provided by human milk, some aspects of her immune system do not fully function on their own for eighteen months, while other aspects take as long as five to six years to fully develop. This timing is not coincidental, as historical and cross-cultural looks at breastfeeding indicate.

A BRIEF HISTORY OF WEANING

In the U.S., babies tend to be weaned young. January 2003 statistics from the U.S. Centers for Disease Control and Prevention tell us that by six months, 66 percent of American babies who started breastfeeding have weaned. By one year, 83 percent have weaned.

But before you make your own decision, we'd like to expand your horizons a little. Our goal in sharing other weaning practices is not to convince you to follow them but to give you a broader perspective on your options. We find it sad that some women wean before they feel ready because others convince them that they are being "selfish" or harming their child by breastfeeding past a certain age. As you will see, what our culture considers normal is at the very early end of the human spectrum. We hope that knowing this will give you more freedom to make your own decisions.

Other times and places. If human societies were viewed as a whole, the average age of weaning would be between two and four years of age. Until the twentieth century, children in both China and Japan breastfed until ages four or five. In 1967, famed anthropologist Margaret Mead and early breastfeeding researcher Niles Newton published an article describing weaning practices of sixty-four traditional cultures. Among all these cultures, only one routinely weaned their children as young as six months.

History tells us that breastfeeding for years was common practice in most times and places. The Koran recommends breastfeeding until age two, and the custom of the Egyptian Pharaohs in Moses's time was to breastfeed for three years. Even in England and the U.S., historical writings tell us that not so long ago two to four years of breastfeeding was typical. In 1725, authors of child-care texts clearly disapproved of four-year-olds breastfeeding, which implies there were more than a few of them around. By 1850, breastfeeding for eleven months was recommended and breastfeeding for two years was criticized. Historically, weaning was considered a dangerous time. In the old West, tombstones of children often listed "weaning death" as the cause (Bumgarner 2000, pp. 80–83).

IS THERE A HUMAN NORM?

In the 1995 book, *Breastfeeding: Biocultural Perspectives*, coeditor Katherine Dettwyler, a cultural anthropologist, attempts to define a biological "human norm" for age of weaning, apart from the influence of culture. To do this, she applied the following criteria, which biologists use to estimate the natural weaning age of other mammals:

- Age at which birth weight is tripled or quadrupled (in humans, two to three years).

- Age at which offspring reach one-third of adult weight (in humans, four to seven years).

- Age of eruption of permanent teeth (in humans, five-and-a-half to six years of age, the same age our immune systems become fully developed).

- Relationship to length of pregnancy (chimpanzees, our nearest relative, breastfeed for six times the length of their pregnancy, which for humans would be four-and-a-half years).

By applying these criteria to humans, she concluded that the natural age of weaning, or the human norm, is between three and seven years.

Are we suggesting that you should breastfeed this long? Not at all. We simply want you to know that *if you decide to breastfeed longer than most people you know, it is not harmful to either you or your child*. On the contrary, as former U.S. Surgeon General Antonia Novello said, "It's the lucky baby, I feel, who continues to nurse until he's two."

Reasons to Wean

There are many reasons women give for weaning, and some of these reasons are entirely justified, while others deserve deeper thought.

REASONS TO THINK TWICE ABOUT WEANING

You may want to think twice if your reason will not accomplish your goal for weaning or if critical information is missing. The following are some of the reasons women wean unnecessarily.

A breastfeeding problem you haven't solved without expert help. A mother in the midst of a breastfeeding crisis often genuinely believes that her situation is hopeless. She may feel as if she has tried everything, even if she hasn't yet sought help from a lactation professional. If you find yourself in this situation, know that a board-certified lactation consultant can most likely offer new strategies you haven't tried. When you have a breastfeeding problem, you need someone both skilled and objective who can help you sort out what is happening and work with you to come up with a solution. Remember, babies are hardwired to breastfeed, and almost all problems are fixable. Don't give up before you've worked with an expert. As we said in the previous chapters, the most common reason given for premature weaning is "worries about milk supply," which is most often due to simple confusion about what's normal.

Return to work. Many mothers manage working and breastfeeding very successfully. Even if you can't express your milk at work, you can still breastfeed when you're home. Some breastfeeding is always better than none. (See the later section, "Partial Weaning," on how to do this. We also provide some more specific strategies in chapter 9.)

One medical opinion. As we'll describe in more detail in the next chapter, we live in a strange world where most health-care professionals have had little to no breastfeeding training or education. This isn't just our opinion. In a survey of 3,115 residents and 1,920 practicing physicians in pediatrics, family practice, and obstetrics, a substantial percentage of respondents gave incorrect responses when asked specific questions about breastfeeding management and seemed unaware of the negative health outcomes of nonhuman milks (Freed et al. 1995a, 1995b).

Yet this lack of knowledge and training doesn't seem to prevent the average physician from giving advice. (One amazing "medical reason" for weaning we've heard lately is "Your baby is allergic to your milk," which is physically impossible.) There are obviously some exceptions to this. We both know physicians who are not only knowledgeable but are leaders in the field. However, if a health-care provider recommends weaning, it's time to get a second opinion. You may want to start by contacting a local lactation consultant or a mother-to-mother breastfeeding counselor for the name of breastfeeding-savvy health-care professionals in your area.

Along these lines, we get many calls from breastfeeding mothers concerned about medications. We'll cover this in more detail in chapter 9. But know now that most drugs are compatible with breastfeeding. Furthermore, in most cases the risks of giving formula are considered to be greater than the risks of taking the drug and continuing to breastfeed. But if you are prescribed one of the rare drugs that is incompatible with breastfeeding, you may still have options. The doctor may be able to substitute another drug. Even if not, you have the option of temporarily weaning, continuing to express your milk, and returning to breastfeeding later.

Mother or baby is ill or hospitalized. This is usually the worst time to wean, as an ill baby will almost always recover faster on human milk. And the last thing an ill or injured mother needs is the pain and health risks of an abrupt weaning (see the last section).

Pregnancy. Some women choose to wean during pregnancy, but you don't have to. There is no evidence that breastfeeding is harmful in any way to the unborn baby.

Baby has teeth. In most places, babies breastfeed long past the age of teething. If biting is a problem for you and your baby, see chapter 10 on ways to stop the biting without weaning.

Baby's on strike. If your baby "weans herself" before one year, chances are it is not a natural weaning but a "nursing strike." If this happens to you, see chapter 10 for ways to get your baby back to breastfeeding.

So baby will sleep better. There is no evidence that weaning (or starting solid foods) helps babies sleep better or longer.

To encourage independence. There is no evidence weaning will do this.

To make your life easier. Weaning is no guarantee of this, either. Once weaned, if your child wakes at night, you now have to get out of bed to settle her down. She is likely to get sick more often. And you will lose the calming and comforting mothering tool of breastfeeding. We don't want you to be disappointed, or worse, find that your life becomes more difficult. Think carefully before weaning for this reason.

YOUR TIME TO WEAN HAS COME

When it's time to wean, be sure you have all the facts, know all your options, and you (or your baby) make the decision to wean. The following reasons indicate your time may have come.

You're ready. You've met your goals or have decided to wean based on your own unique considerations. Or you've simply decided the time is right.

Your child's ready. As Law 7 says, all children will eventually wean naturally (see the upcoming section "Natural Weaning"), sometimes even before their mothers are ready to wean. Natural weaning can happen as young as twelve months.

A confirmed medical issue. By "confirmed" we mean you've gotten a second opinion, as well as spoken to a lactation consultant. Many mothers wean unnecessarily on the recommendation of a health-care provider who later proves to be wrong. Two medically valid reasons to wean involving mother's health include chemotherapy for cancer or radioactive therapy for thyroid problems.

OTHER REASONS TO WEAN

Some reasons to wean can be trickier to negotiate and deserve some extra thought.

Feeling overwhelmed with breastfeeding. If this is your reason, we hope you have sought skilled breastfeeding help. Often there are ways to make breastfeeding easier. But there are some situations, for example, mothers with a history of childhood sexual abuse, in which breastfeeding can feel overwhelming even when it's going well. If you do feel overwhelmed, you still have options. Women who have difficulty with the close body contact of breastfeeding sometimes pump their milk and give it to their baby by bottle. Some do a partial weaning, eliminating breastfeedings until they feel more at ease. Some breastfeeding is always better than none. See chapter 10 for more suggestions.

Social or family pressures. Some women find themselves in a family or an environment in which breastfeeding is frowned upon. It takes a strong person to breastfeed in spite of an unsupportive partner, family, or social circle. If this is your problem, consider finding the support you need elsewhere. In one study, mother-to-mother support was essential to maintaining breastfeeding when mothers were feeling pressured to wean. Family members and strangers were the two groups of people most likely to be critical of mothers who breastfed for longer than six months (Kendall-Tackett and Sugarman 1995). Many mothers attend weekly mothers' meetings at their hospital, monthly mother-to-mother breastfeeding groups (for example, La Leche League, Nursing Mothers Counsel, Australian Breastfeeding Association), or both, as an antidote to the negativity they face in the wider world. Meeting with other like-minded women—even once a month—can make a tremendous difference.

WHAT MOTHERS SAY ABOUT WEANING

Your feelings are an important part of the weaning equation. If you are considering weaning because you find breastfeeding stressful, it may help to know what mothers say about weaning with the benefit of hindsight. In one 1987 study, Cosby Rogers and his colleagues asked women their feelings about weaning well after the fact and found that 65 percent who weaned their babies at three months or younger had regrets. More than 50 percent of those who weaned at four to six months wished they had breastfed longer. Norma Jane Bumgarner, author of *Mothering Your Nursing Toddler* (2000), a book for those who breastfeed past one year, noted after reading letters from hundreds of mothers that those who most consistently described feelings of loss and regret after weaning were those who weaned before two years.

> When nursing continues past two or three, mothers much less frequently describe weaning in the same mixed terms. It seems that a time comes in the growth of the mother-child relationship when it is easier for both to move on and leave baby things behind. (Bumgarner 2000, p. 288)

If you are considering weaning before you had intended because of mixed or negative feelings, you owe it to both your baby and yourself to talk to a breastfeeding professional to see if there is a solution or adjustment that would help you feel better about continuing.

WEANING BASICS

When your time comes to wean, remember Law 7: "Children wean naturally." We hope that this, along with the following information, will help you navigate this inevitable transition comfortably and happily.

Ideally, weaning should always be done gradually. Unfortunately, gradual weaning runs counter to the most commonly given advice, which is to stop breastfeeding abruptly, bind the breasts, and wait for the pain to subside. This is a barbaric approach that is unnecessarily painful and risky.

To appreciate why, consider the alternative. If weaning is gradual enough, you will never feel pain or discomfort. You will also avoid health risks, which include a painful complication that could require hospitalization and surgery (see the last section for more on this). For your baby, a gradual weaning gives you time to make sure she tolerates well whatever formula or other food you substitute before your milk is gone. A gradual weaning also allows you to give your baby more focused attention and comforting skin-to-skin contact to make the emotional adjustment easier for her. Since breastfeeding is a part of your close relationship, you want your baby to know that you are not withdrawing your love along with your breasts.

Approaches to Weaning

As we said at the beginning, your approach to weaning makes all the difference. Let's take a closer look at some of your choices and how they work.

REDUCING MILK SUPPLY COMFORTABLY

As you wean, your goal is to reduce your milk supply gradually and comfortably. To do this, let's apply what we learned in chapter 6 in reverse. As we explained, milk supply is determined by the number of times per day milk is drained from the breasts and how much milk is drained, either by a baby or by pumping. So to decrease your milk supply gradually, you can do one or both of the following:

- Gradually decrease the amount of milk drained from the breasts each time.

- Gradually decrease the number of times per day the breasts are drained.

However, as with many things in life, the devil is in the details. The following sections describe different approaches to weaning and how these principles apply.

NATURAL WEANING

Let's start with the approach that most U.S. mothers seem to know the least about, but when considered within the big picture of human history, may be the most commonly used. This is to allow your baby to outgrow breastfeeding, otherwise known as "natural weaning."

Why some choose natural weaning. Even in the U.S., where 83 percent of babies are weaned by one year, some mothers choose natural weaning. Some choose it because it feels right to them. Others because it allows their child to grow at her own pace and wean according to her own inner timetable. Still others choose natural weaning because it is the least work.

Although the uninitiated sometimes assume that breastfeeding past one year is an act of martyrdom, mothers report that in many ways breastfeeding a toddler makes their lives easier. The relaxing breastfeeding hormones help mothers keep their cool, even under duress. And as a mothering tool, breastfeeding continues to make naptimes and bedtimes blissfully easy as well as ending tantrums in the blink of an eye.

Natural weaning is usually gradual, although an occasional toddler may naturally wean earlier and more abruptly than her mother expects. More commonly, though, your milk supply reduces slowly and comfortably without any thought or effort as your child's attention becomes more focused on the world around her and less on you. Another plus of natural weaning is that you never have to deal with an unhappy child resisting your efforts to wean or the hassle of weaning from the bottle later. As one mother said, "I wouldn't think of limiting or ending the breastfeeding relationship any more than I would think of limiting or ending my love for my children. Gradual weaning allowed us both to grow into other ways of expressing our love" (Kendall-Tackett and Sugarman 1995, p. 181). Many women who wean naturally report that

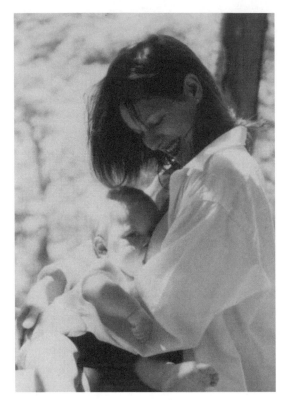

Breastfeeding provides comfort and emotional security to older babies as they venture into the wider world. (©2005 Mary Jane Chase, RNC, MN, CCE, IBCLC, used with permission)

the process was so gradual that they are not even sure when their child's last breastfeeding happened.

At what age do children naturally wean? Many mothers worry that if they don't take the lead in weaning that their child will breastfeed "forever." In reality, all children outgrow breastfeeding. How long does it take? It varies from child to child, like the age they learn to walk, talk, and get their first tooth. One child may wean at one or two years while another may be avidly breastfeeding at three. A child with a strong sucking urge, an intense need for closeness, or an unrecognized allergy or other physical problem may breastfeed longer than others.

Social challenges. As we described earlier, one study (Kendall-Tackett and Sugarman 1995) found that for many U.S. mothers, the biggest challenge of natural weaning is coping with others' opinions, and the older the child, the more challenging this becomes. Yet, in spite of this, the study mothers felt that the positives outweighed the negatives.

One way to handle social challenges is to keep breastfeeding private. This is an option because an older child does not usually breastfeed as often as a young baby. Some tried-and-true strategies for avoiding breastfeeding in a less-than-friendly environment include:

- setting limits on where and when your child can breastfeed;

- bringing snacks, drinks, toys, and/or books to distract your child when you go out;

- choosing a "code word" for breastfeeding that won't be obvious to others;

- finding private places to breastfeed outside the home, such as fitting rooms or "mothers' lounges" at the mall;

- carefully choosing your clothing. Two-piece outfits are best. Cover-ups like ponchos or shawls can help, too.

The importance of support. Mothers who breastfeed longer than their cultural norm enjoy the experience more if they have support. Mother-to-mother breastfeeding groups like La Leche League, Nursing Mothers Counsel, and the Australian Breastfeeding Association are great places to meet others who value breastfeeding at all ages.

PLANNED WEANING AFTER ONE YEAR

Let's say your goal is to breastfeed for one or two years, but you prefer to wean before your child outgrows breastfeeding. If so, this section is for you.

Even though the child one year or older may have strong preferences about breastfeeding—as she will about all aspects of her daily routine—you can still make weaning a gradual and positive experience. To accomplish this, first allow plenty of time. It may take several weeks to wean, depending on how many times a day she has been breastfeeding. You also need to consider her temperament and opinions, and factor them into your strategies. Think about alternatives that she might consider even better than breastfeeding, because, as author and pediatrician Dr. William Sears says, "A wise baby who enjoys a happy nursing relationship is not likely to give it up willingly unless some other form of emotional nourishment is provided that is equally attractive or at least interestingly different" (cited in Mohrbacher 1995). The following strategies are among your many options:

Don't offer, don't refuse. Breastfeed when she asks but otherwise don't offer. When used with other strategies, this one can speed up the process.

Offer regular meals, snacks, and drinks. Minimize her hunger and thirst with alternatives to breastfeeding, and offer her age-appropriate fun activities to avoid breastfeeding out of boredom.

Change daily routines. Think about the times and places she asks to breastfeed and how to change your routine so she will be reminded less often. For example, if she usually asks to breastfeed when you sit in a certain chair, avoid that chair.

Get your partner involved. If she usually breastfeeds first thing in the morning, ask your partner to get her up and give her breakfast. Your partner can also help her get back to sleep when she wakes at night and plan special daytime outings together to distract her from her usual routine.

Anticipate and offer substitutes and distractions. Be sure to offer substitutes *before* she asks to breastfeed, because once she's asked, she will likely feel rejected and upset if a substitute is offered. As an example, right before a usual breastfeeding time offer a special snack and drink and then take her to a favorite place, such as a playground, as a distraction. Some children breastfeed more often at home with nothing to do and less when out and distracted. For this type of child, spend as much of the day as possible out of the house. Other children breastfeed more often when in new surroundings. For a child like this, stay home more and keep distractions to a minimum.

Postpone. This works for a child who breastfeeds at irregular times and places and is old enough to accept waiting. If postponing leaves your child feeling as though you are keeping her at arm's length, she may become even more determined to breastfeed. If so, use other strategies.

Shorten the length of breastfeedings. This is most effective with children older than two and is a good beginning to the weaning process.

Bargaining. This one can work well with the older child. A child who is close to outgrowing breastfeeding may give up breastfeeding earlier by mutual agreement. But most children younger than three do not have the maturity and perspective to understand the meaning of a promise.

Adjust your plan based on your child's reactions and preferences. Pick and choose among these strategies based on your child's reactions. One child may be unhappy with postponing but do well with distraction and substitution. Also, certain breastfeedings may be more important to your child than others. If so, continue those until the end and allow your child to give them up last. If she clings to these breastfeedings, you can continue with them for a while. Often the bedtime breastfeeding is a favorite.

Be flexible. When unusual situations arise, avoid sticking rigidly to your weaning strategies. If your child is ill, she may want to breastfeed more often for comfort. You can go back to weaning after she's feeling better.

When to slow down. Even at the same age, some children will be more ready to wean than others. If your child becomes upset and cries or insists upon breastfeeding even when you try to distract or comfort her in others ways, this may mean that weaning is going too fast for her or that different strategies would be better. Other signs that weaning may be moving too fast are changes or regressions in behavior, such as stuttering, night-waking, an increase in clinginess, a new or increased fear of separation, biting (if she has never bitten before), stomach upsets, and constipation.

Make weaning a positive experience for your child by paying attention to your own inner voice and being sensitive to your child's cues.

PLANNED WEANING OF A YOUNGER BABY

When weaning a child younger than one year, the nutritional aspects of breastfeeding need to be considered first. So before beginning weaning, consult your baby's health-care provider for recommendations for human milk substitutes. The feeding method you choose will depend upon your baby's age. If she is close to a year old and drinking well from a cup, you may be able to forego the bottle entirely and go directly to a cup, which avoids the need to wean again from a bottle later.

The practical details of weaning. If she is much younger than twelve months, you'll need to substitute some type of formula for breastfeeding, as regular cow's milk is not recommended until after one year. Here's how to wean step by step at this stage:

- First, make note of the times you usually breastfeed.

- Pick one daily breastfeeding (leave the first morning breast-feeding for last) and instead substitute formula by bottle (or cup, for the older baby).

- Give your body at least two to three days to adjust before dropping another breastfeeding so that your milk supply has time to decrease comfortably and gradually.

- If at any time your breasts feel full, express just enough milk to feel comfortable (pump just to comfort—no longer) or allow the baby to breastfeed for a short time. *There are health risks to allowing your breasts to get or stay uncomfortably full.* Pay attention to your body's cues, expressing milk to comfort whenever needed.

Following this plan, it usually takes about two to three weeks to go from exclusive breastfeeding to a complete weaning.

When you're down to breastfeeding just once or twice a day, if there is no rush to wean completely, you can continue these breast-feedings for as long as you like. Your breasts will continue to produce enough milk as long as your baby breastfeeds. Remember, some breast-feeding is always better than none.

The importance of reassurance. A gradual weaning like this gives you time to make sure your baby is adjusting well to the change and to give her extra focused and loving attention as a substitute for the closeness you shared while breastfeeding.

Other outlets for sucking. Because babies come hardwired with a strong need to suck until the natural age of weaning, they may find another outlet, such as thumbsucking, during or after weaning. If you prefer your baby use a bottle or pacifier, you can offer one of these instead.

PARTIAL WEANING

This can be an alternative to total weaning for the mother who finds the body contact of breastfeeding difficult or some other aspect of breastfeeding either impractical or overwhelming. It can also be a compromise for the mother returning to work who doesn't plan to express her milk while away from her baby. A partial weaning can allow her to continue breastfeeding when she's home and yet bring her milk supply down to the point where she doesn't have to pump at work.

To do a partial weaning, follow the step-by-step instructions in the previous section to decrease your number of breastfeedings until your milk supply adjusts gradually downward. Once you have reached the point that your breasts do not get uncomfortably full for the length of time you're away from your baby, you can continue with that number of breastfeedings. Once there, you can continue breastfeeding at this level indefinitely.

ABRUPT WEANING

Although this is the least desirable of your options, it is sometimes necessary in cases of tragedy (the death of a baby) or a medical emergency. If abrupt weaning is necessary, first consider your options, get a second opinion, and talk to a lactation consultant. Many times there are alternatives to weaning you may be unaware of. If an abrupt weaning is unavoidable:

- Wear a firm bra for support (one size larger than usual so it does not get too tight).

- Reduce your salt intake but not your fluids.

- Express enough milk as needed to stay comfortable.

To wean quickly, use an effective breast pump (such as a rental pump) to make the process as gradual and comfortable as possible. As your milk supply decreases, the need to express milk also decreases. Remember, *do not wait to express milk until you are overly full or in pain. There are health risks to unrelieved breast fullness.* (See the final section of this chapter.)

Attend to your baby's emotional needs. An abrupt weaning is the most stressful for you and your baby. No matter what her age, breast-feeding is part of her close relationship with you. Keep this in mind and be sure baby gets lots of focused attention and skin-to-skin contact to reassure her that you have not withdrawn your love. If you are not available, be sure your baby has someone else to hold and comfort her.

The Role of Solid Foods

Depending on the age of your child, the introduction of solid foods may play a significant role in the weaning process.

SOLIDS AND MILK SUPPLY

An important point to know is that when solid foods are introduced, they do not increase a baby's overall intake. Solids take the place of your milk or formula in your baby's diet. If you are exclusively breastfeeding, this changes the equation that determines your milk supply. In chapter 6, we described how milk supply is based on the number of times per day your breasts are drained and how well they are drained. As your baby takes more solids, she takes less milk. This is why your timing and strategy for giving solid foods can affect your long-term breastfeeding goals.

WHEN TO START SOLIDS

A generation ago, mothers were encouraged to give their babies solids within the first six weeks. But as the practice of early solids was studied, researchers found serious drawbacks for both mothers and babies and this practice was abandoned. As we mentioned in the preceding chapter, the still-common recommendation of starting solid foods at four to six months is now being revised. In 2001, the World Health Organization's panel of experts examined the available research on the ideal age for starting solids and concluded that waiting to start solids for a full six months results in better health outcomes for mothers and babies. Because a younger baby's digestive system is not yet mature enough to handle solid foods well, babies who start solids before six months are at higher risk for:

- Allergies

- Ear infections

- Digestive problems

When solids are given too early, a more age-appropriate food is replaced with a food that she cannot yet fully digest. But because solid foods fill her up and make her less interested in breastfeeding, the earlier solids are started, the greater the risk that a mother's milk supply will be reduced before she is ready to wean.

Baby's signs of readiness. On a practical level, giving solids to babies younger than six months is difficult, because babies are born with a tongue-thrust reflex that causes them to push out with their tongue anything that goes into their mouth. This tongue thrusting, which is usually outgrown between four and six months, makes feeding a young baby solids an exercise in frustration.

What we're beginning to understand is that physical readiness for solids coincides with your baby's ability to feed herself, which makes good, logical sense. Your baby is most likely ready for solids when she reaches this level of maturity and you see the following signs of readiness:

- She can sit up alone.

- She can pick up food and put it in her mouth.

- Her tongue-thrust reflex has disappeared.

- She shows an interest in eating other foods.

This last point is crucial, as experience has shown that babies who are at risk for allergies tend to refuse solids until they are a little older, possibly in an effort to protect their sensitive digestive systems. So if a baby does not want solids exactly at six months, it is best to continue to offer them about once a week, but to let your baby take the lead.

Signs to ignore. The following are *not* indicators of a baby's readiness for solids:

- Baby reaches a certain weight (despite what commercial baby food companies say).

- Baby is not sleeping well at night (see the later section "Solids and Sleep" on this).

HOW TO START SOLIDS

Keep in mind that between six months and nine months or so, your baby needs your milk more than she needs solid foods. This means that the amount of solid foods she takes is less important than the practice she's getting. Think of this as a time when she learns to eat solids before they really matter to her nutritionally.

One food at a time, and start small. Give single foods at first rather than mixtures. Allow at least a week between new foods, so you will know if she reacts to a particular food. Begin by giving a small amount at a time (maybe ¼ tsp or about 1 ml), increasing the amount over the week before another food is offered. Once she has done well with several foods, feel free to mix them.

Signs of food sensitivity. The following are signs a baby is reacting badly to a food:

- Hives, diaper rash, or eczema

- Runny nose or congestion

- Wheezing

- Red, itchy eyes

- Ear infection

- Fussiness

- Digestive problems—constipation, vomiting, diarrhea

If you see any of these signs, eliminate that food and try it again next week. If baby reacts again, avoid it for several months.

No need to puree. For the baby six months or older, it is not necessary to puree foods. Just use a fork to mash and moisten the foods you and your family are eating before salt, sugar, and spices are added. (For the exceptions, see "Solids to avoid until one year" in this section.)

Expect messes. Allow your baby to feed herself and play with the food. This can be messy, so use bibs, undress baby to a diaper, bathe after feedings, and/or put plastic down around baby's chair. Let your baby experience food with all her senses and decide how much food *she* wants to eat. This promotes healthy eating habits.

Foods to choose. The foods given to babies when they start solids vary around the world depending on the locale, the culture, the season, and the foods available. When deciding on a food for your baby, keep in mind that fresh foods are more nutritious than processed foods. Some of the fresh foods you can choose include ripe, mashed banana, cooked sweet potato or yam, ripe avocado, tender stewed or ground meat or poultry mashed and moistened, tofu, cooked rice or oats, boiled or baked peeled white potato, grated apple or applesauce, ripe peach, pear, apricots, cooked carrots, frozen peas, and egg yolks.

Solids to avoid until one year. Foods best avoided until a baby is one year old include cow's milk, egg whites, peanuts, citrus fruits, shellfish, honey (due to botulism spores), and any food of a size and shape that might block baby's windpipe, such as hot dogs and raw carrots (until three years).

Solids to avoid in allergic families. If you have a family history of allergies, other foods to consider delaying until one year are wheat, corn, pork, fish, tomatoes, onions, cabbage, berries, nuts, and spices.

SOLIDS AND SLEEP

Many parents are anxious to start solid foods because they've heard that their babies will sleep better. However, two studies that monitored babies' sleep habits found no correlation between solid foods and sleep (Macknin et al. 1989; Keane et al. 1988). The same number of babies who hadn't yet started solids slept through the night as those who were given rice cereal right before bed. In their 1989 study, Michael Macknin and his colleagues concluded that ". . . infants' ability to sleep through the night is a developmental and adaptive process that occurs regardless of the timing of introduction of cereal" (p. 1068).

WHEN THE SYSTEM BREAKS DOWN

Throughout this chapter we have alluded to the risks of abrupt weaning. Now it's time to get more specific. If you ever find yourself in a situation in which abrupt weaning is recommended, as we've said, it is wise to get a second opinion and talk to a lactation consultant, because other options can usually be found.

Risks of Abrupt Weaning

Unfortunately, when a mother asks how to wean, abrupt weaning is often the first and only approach she is given. Many health-care providers tell mothers to simply stop breastfeeding, bind their breasts, and wait until the pain subsides. (That's easy for them to say!) This is an unnecessarily stressful and risky way to wean. Now let's examine why.

RISKS OF ABRUPT WEANING TO YOU

The physical risks of a sudden weaning are the most obvious and are reason enough to take a gradual approach.

Pain. When a mother stops breastfeeding suddenly, her breasts continue making milk. When the milk is not removed, her breasts first become full, fuller, overly full, and then painfully engorged. Some women describe the pain they've suffered with abrupt weaning as the worst pain they've ever experienced. We've received frantic calls from weaning mothers in pain who ask what to do to relieve it. "Breastfeed or pump" is our usual reply. There's no reason in the world to endure this pain when weaning can be done comfortably and gradually.

Mastitis. Unrelieved breast fullness is one cause of *mastitis*, which is an inflammation of the breasts. Mastitis can be mild or severe and covers a spectrum of symptoms. We describe it in more detail in chapter 10.

Mild mastitis, or "plugged ducts," are sore, lumpy areas in the breast. They are usually easily treated, but if the milk is not removed well and often, it can progress to a more severe form, in which the sore areas become red and hot and the mother develops a fever and flu-like symptoms. The best treatment for mastitis is frequent breast drainage, either by breastfeeding (which is preferred) or by breast pumping, along with warm compresses and rest. But if a mother with mastitis is weaning (not recommended!) and she does not drain the milk from her breasts often, the condition can worsen. If her breast fullness is unrelieved and her mastitis with fever is not treated quickly with the right antibiotics, the condition can progress into its most severe form, breast abscess.

Breast abscess. A breast abscess is a walled-off, pus-filled area within the breast. When a mother develops this complication, which happens in 5 to 11 percent of women with infectious mastitis who receive incorrect or delayed treatment, she may need to be hospitalized and the abscess drained surgically. Due to this risk, weaning is never recommended during mastitis. See chapter 10 for more information on mastitis.

Emotional distress. Women who have been forced to wean before they are ready often speak of the sadness and despair they felt. They grieve the loss of breastfeeding and its special closeness.

RISKS OF ABRUPT WEANING TO YOUR BABY

When breastfeeding is withdrawn suddenly, a baby can also have physical and emotional reactions.

Reactions to alternative foods. A baby who is allergic or sensitive to nonhuman milks or other foods may have a strong physical reaction when breastfeeding is withdrawn suddenly and her system is flooded with triggering foods (for specifics, see the possible reactions to solids listed in the earlier section). A gradual weaning allows a mother to determine her baby's tolerance of other foods before moving forward. It also gives her time to reconsider if her baby doesn't handle the alternatives well.

Emotional distress. Because breastfeeding is a source of comfort and closeness as well as food, an abrupt weaning is emotionally stressful. If you have no choice but to wean abruptly, make every effort to give your baby lots of reassurance, focused attention, and skin-to-skin contact.

SUMMARY

Weaning need not be a painful process for you or your baby. For your and baby's sake, avoid abrupt weaning if at all possible. You can choose to allow your child to wean naturally. Or, if you choose to take the lead, going slowly will help, you avoid the possible physical and emotional complications that can occur, and you give yourself time to evaluate how well your baby is adapting to weaning. By waiting until your child is ready or by easing off breastfeeding gradually and expressing your love in other ways, weaning can be a joyful celebration of your child's coming of age, or at the very least, a positive experience for both of you.

CHAPTER 8

What Interferes with the Laws

In the last seven chapters, we've described how simple breastfeeding can be and how important it is to the health of mothers and babies. If what we say is true, then you might wonder how our culture managed to stray so far from breastfeeding as the biological norm for you and your baby. That's the focus of this chapter. To answer this question, we must take you on a brief excursion through history. Understanding how we got to this point is important since much of the bad breastfeeding advice that you will receive stems from specific historical and cultural movements and their related beliefs. If you know where various ideas came from, you'll be in a much better position to evaluate them and decide whether they will work for you and your family. Here we go.

THE ROLE OF HISTORY AND CULTURE

To understand where we are now, we need to go back in time more than 150 years. In the U.S. and other parts of the world, the Industrial

Revolution was in full swing. As a wider variety of mass-produced products became available, people's standards of living began to rise. Innovation was equated with improvement in everyday comfort. Products that we all now take for granted, like reliable sources of heat and light and indoor plumbing, were widely available for the first time to ordinary people. The amount of change that families experienced during this time was unprecedented. It seemed like every day brought a new innovation that made problems that people had dealt with for millennia suddenly disappear. The old ways of doing things suddenly seemed out of place in the new technological age.

Science was also making significant advances, most notably in its battle against disease. Problems that had terrorized people for thousands of years were overcome. There was the advent of anesthesia, which allowed doctors to operate without killing their patients from shock. There was effective pain relief. There was the germ theory of infection. Mortality rates dropped. It was a heady time. Science seemed to hold the promise of eradicating all human misery. Many traditional methods of health and healing were seen as out of step with the new science.

The Rise of Scientific Mothering

It wasn't long before the lens of science and technology was turned upon mothers and babies. Soon, scientists pronounced that the only proper way to raise a baby was with "scientific mothering." Parenting manuals became popular during this time, so that male experts could share with mothers the "latest techniques." Mothers were advised not to spoil their babies with affection, to provide them a clean and sterile environment, and to use a strict schedule for everything from eating, to sleeping, to toilet training.

FEEDING BY THE CLOCK

One of the beliefs that grew out of the scientific-mothering approach was that babies should be fed at predetermined intervals. The clock, rather than the baby's sense of hunger, should determine when babies were next fed. We are still dealing with the impact of this mistaken belief today.

You can see how breastfeeding would be unappealing to those who adopted this regularized and "scientific" approach to raising children. Breastfeeding is more intuitive, relying upon mothers being able to read their babies cues. Mothers and babies determine when the baby has had enough, rather than outside experts. The whole process of breastfeeding seemed sloppy and messy and completely unscientific.

NONHUMAN MILKS

It was against this backdrop that man-made baby milks first became widely commercially available and gained broad acceptance. In this era of scientific mothering, these products—called "formula" in reference to their scientific origins—were actually touted as being *better* for babies than their mothers' milk.

Prior to this time, people had experimented with all manner of substitutes for human milk, and, unfortunately, in most places a high rate of infant mortality resulted. Some examples of food given to babies were beer, "sops" (bread soaked in milk or water), and gruel (cereal). It's a wonder that any survived this kind of regimen. Babies of wealthy families were also often put out to "wet-nurse" with other women who were hired to feed the babies. Even with breastfeeding, many of these babies died—perhaps due to neglect of wet nurses who were caring for too many babies at once (it was said that wet nurses were "limited" to six babies at a time).

Around the same time that nonhuman baby milks became commercially available, pediatrics, a new medical specialty, came into existence. Mothers were told that rather than using family-practice doctors, as before, they should take their babies to the new "baby doctors," because they were trained to create "formulas" to meet each baby's individual needs. (For more information on the history of this era and the ties between pediatrics and the formula industry, see the book *The Politics of Breastfeeding* by Gabrielle Palmer.) Formula also appealed to a science-enamored generation because it was easy to tell just how many ounces a baby was taking. Therefore, feeding could be regulated and monitored in a precise way. It sounded like a great system—except for the fact that babies were dying.

The price of progress. As early as the 1920s, researchers found that babies fed with these nonhuman milks had a mortality rate of three to six times higher than their breastfed counterparts (Woodbury 1925). And that was in the U.S. The picture was far bleaker in the developing world, and it still is today.

Unethical marketing practices. As the decades passed and their products became widely used in developed countries like the U.S., formula companies realized that developing nations were also a potentially lucrative market. In a shameful chapter in the history of this industry, women were hired to dress like nurses and offer free samples of formula to mothers—just enough so that their milk supply would decrease or disappear. Then women thought they had no choice but to continue to buy formula, even when they couldn't afford it, even when they had to mix it with contaminated water. The irresponsibility of these multinational corporations led to worldwide boycotts of their products. The death rate was staggeringly high, and finally led the World Health Organization to take steps to limit how formula companies could market their products. This is known as the WHO International Code of Marketing of Breast-Milk Substitutes, or the "WHO Code" for short. The U.S. as a country does not adhere to the WHO Code, but some U.S. organizations do.

Just as good? Unfortunately, there are still problems today. Formula has gained a solid place among mothers around the world who are being told that nonhuman milks are "just as good" as human milk and that bottle feeding is the "modern" way to feed a baby. Unfortunately, women coming to the U.S. from developing countries often abandon breastfeeding in favor of more "modern" ways of feeding their babies, even if they breastfed their children in their home countries. And many women born in the U.S. (including many health professionals) are unaware of the health consequences to them and to their babies if they don't breastfeed. So when these women have breastfeeding difficulties, they are more likely to give up.

WILL THE REAL SCIENTIFIC MOTHER PLEASE STAND UP?

In retrospect, we see that the efficacy of science was vastly overestimated. Science did not bring an end to all human suffering. Just when one problem was conquered, another reared its ugly head. For example, when smallpox was virtually eliminated, scientists were then faced with the AIDS epidemic, which shows no sign of slowing down. And even smallpox is reappearing. It was, in many cases, pure hubris to suggest that science could create a perfect world.

Losing the human touch. We are also realizing now that we were too quick to abandon many of the old ways that were actually quite effective and indeed probably better than what replaced them. In medicine, there are numerous examples of this. In recent times, patients started to protest what seemed to them to be a purely mechanistic approach to health and healing. They wanted to be treated as whole people, not just the sum of body parts. One example of this reaction is the astounding growth of alternative medicine, with herbal medicine being the most visible example. Another example is the burgeoning field of health psychology, where research has found that people's attitudes, beliefs, and social connections are important to survival.

Breastfeeding and survival. Interestingly, science has also come around to the breastfeeding point of view. As we explained in the introduction, thousands of studies have now demonstrated the inferiority of nonhuman milks when compared with breastfeeding. The women who defied the "wisdom" of their day and breastfed their babies were in fact the *real scientific* mothers, and we are in their debt. These were the mothers who paid attention to their babies' cues, who fed the babies when they were hungry, rocked or carried them when they were cranky, and came to them when they cried. They ignored the experts and listened to their own hearts. On the surface, their approach seems the exact opposite of scientific. But if scientific means increasing the likelihood that their babies would survive, then they were right on the money.

Cultural Beliefs About Babies and Breastfeeding

Despite the amply-demonstrated inferiority of nonhuman milks to breastfeeding, scientific mothering is still alive and well. Many of our cultural beliefs that undermine breastfeeding are an outgrowth of both scientific mothering and generations of bottle feeding. There are many misconceptions about the needs of babies that are prominent in our culture, even though science has soundly disproved them. Here are a few of the beliefs that can be destructive to you and your baby. Know that these have no scientific support despite the widespread belief to the contrary.

THE IMPORTANCE OF SCHEDULE

As a new mother, the most common questions people will ask you are whether your baby is sleeping through the night and on some type of regular eating and sleeping schedule. These are purported to be "good" characteristics, while nonregulated eating and sleeping patterns are "bad."

These beliefs about the importance of schedule are based on a couple of erroneous assumptions. First, they assume that all mothers and babies are the same, which they are not (see chapter 6). Second, they fail to take into account babies' legitimate physical needs, such as hunger. As we described in chapter 4, a newborn baby has a stomach the size of a marble. Your baby is in the best position to tell you whether he is hungry. The use of "ideal feeding schedules" has abso- lutely no basis in science. That bears saying again: *there is no science that supports a feeding schedule for a breastfed baby.* When a schedule becomes your principle guide about when to feed your baby, you are no longer reading your baby's feeding cues. The net result is that your baby's instinctive feeding behavior is suppressed. Both you and your baby lose.

THE PARENT MUST BE THE BOSS

This is another belief that we frequently hear from mothers, and it saddens us. This belief often has religious overtones that gravely warn parents to "discipline" their children from the start lest they lose control. You don't want your child to grow up to be a drug addict, do you? This belief depends heavily on some pretty weak logic. We agree that disciplining children is part of the responsibility of parents. No question. But it is absurd to extrapolate that belief into thinking that by feeding your child when he's hungry—especially if he's an infant— you are somehow giving in to your child and making him "willful." A baby who cries when he is hungry is expressing a legitimate physical need, a need that ensures his survival. By crying, a baby is commu- nicating in his most direct and attention-getting way. In terms of how "giving in" to babies sets them up for future behavior problems, science has found that the opposite is true. Babies reared by nonresponsive or harsh parents are significantly more likely to engage in harmful behaviors—including drug abuse. This has been repeatedly demonstrated in dozens of studies. Bottom line: responding to your baby's needs is good for him.

BABIES MANIPULATE ADULTS BY CRYING

This belief is similar to the one described above. It is something, sadly, that we hear from mothers on a regular basis. Mothers often believe that they shouldn't "give in" to their babies because that would be doing what the babies want. Yes, that's precisely it! Remember, crying and fussing are the only ways babies can communicate. Telling you that they want to be fed, changed, or held is perfectly legitimate. It is not manipulative for your baby to tell you that he needs something that will allow him to survive.

You can consider this question another way. Is your baby sophisticated enough to manipulate you? To do this, babies must form what developmental psychologists call a *meta-cognition*. That is, they must be able to think about what they are thinking ("If I cry, then someone will come"). Babies can't do this until they are many months old. They can't yet conceive of the results of their actions. They just know they need help.

IGNORING A BABY'S CRIES WILL MAKE HIM CRY LESS

This belief maintains that if you want a baby who cries less, you should not respond to his cries, and it is straight out of the philosophy of behaviorism. Back in its heyday, behaviorists such as John B. Watson told mothers not to hold, touch, or cuddle their babies for fear of spoiling them. Behaviorism is one of the schools of thought that brought us scientific mothering. Some vestiges of this belief still exist today. In fact, you may be surprised to learn that many students of psychology are still taught this both as graduate students and as undergraduates. Again, this is one of those beliefs that doesn't stand up to scientific scrutiny.

In the U.S., longitudinal studies have compared mothers who are responsive to their babies during infancy and mothers who were less responsive. The burning question was: If mothers ignored their babies' cries, would the babies cry less than babies of mothers who responded promptly? Guess what! The responsive mothers had babies who cried less (Bates, Maslin, and Frankel 1985; Crockenberg and McCluskey 1986).

The importance of responsive parenting has also been demonstrated in cross-cultural research. Research into other cultures is valuable because researchers are often unaware of the values, beliefs, and assumptions that they bring to their research. For example, in the not-too-distant past, it was difficult to study breastfeeding mothers in this culture because they were such a small minority of women. Many of the standards we use to measure normal infant development (such as growth charts) are based on babies who were formula fed. That is changing, but it goes to show how pervasive the influence of culture is. When researchers went into completely different cultures, many of the things researchers believed were normal were quickly exposed as being part of their culture, not universal human traits. You might be surprised to learn that not all human babies regularly cry. That's what research on a tribe called the !Kung found.

The !Kung are a traditional culture and tribe who are considered hunter-gatherers. It has been instructive for many to observe their childrearing strategies. In this culture, babies sleep with their mothers. They are held most of the time, since there is no safe place to set them down. Their mothers often wear them by placing them in a carrier on their bodies, where the babies have near constant access to their mothers' breasts and breastfeed at will. And they rarely cry. As toddlers, these babies are *more* independent than their counterparts in the U.S. (Konner 1976).

This is just one of many examples in the literature. When studying other cultures, we don't want to assume that they do everything better than we do. Nor do we want to reject what they do as being too "primitive." But these other cultures can be instructive—especially because they haven't been touched by industrialization and scientific mothering. So many tenets of that approach have been refuted that any advice based on that approach bears close scrutiny.

Unfortunately, scientific mothering is not the only cultural force that can interfere with breastfeeding.

General Ignorance of Breastfeeding

Ignorance is another influential force undermining the natural laws of breastfeeding. An obvious consequence of this ignorance, combined with poor breastfeeding management, is the sharp drop-off of exclusive breastfeeding after birth. According to the U.S. Centers for Disease Control and Prevention, in January 2003 62 percent of U.S. mothers were exclusively breastfeeding at one week, but by four months, that number dropped to 30 percent.

Ignorance about breastfeeding has its roots in our familiarity with bottlefeeding. As we have explained, breastfeeding is best learned by watching others do it as a normal part of daily life. On the other hand, those of us who grew up exposed primarily to bottlefeeding have bottle-feeding "norms" ingrained in our thinking, consciously or unconsciously, and these expectations may need to be unlearned.

APPLYING BOTTLE-FEEDING NORMS

Many women approach breastfeeding thinking, either consciously or subconsciously, that they can use what they know about bottle feeding to breastfeed. Unfortunately, there are enough basic differences that this does not usually work well.

Using bottle-feeding technique to breastfeed. As an example, in the early 1980s, many mothers were instructed to hold their babies in their arms for breastfeeding with their babies facing the ceiling (a bottle-feeding position). They were then told to tickle the baby's cheek with their nipple until baby turned his head toward the breast and then to let the baby latch on. To understand how difficult it is to feed in this position, try turning your head all the way to one side and swallow. Using a bottle-feeding position to breastfeed made it difficult for a baby and was no doubt one factor contributing to the common misconception that nipple trauma is normal for breastfeeding mothers. (Not so!) When babies fed with their heads turned, they pulled on the nipple, causing pain and trauma.

As we'll explain more fully in the last section of this chapter, health-care providers often have poor or outdated information about breastfeeding. This means that the people new mothers tend to turn to first, doctors and nurses, usually know little about how to manage

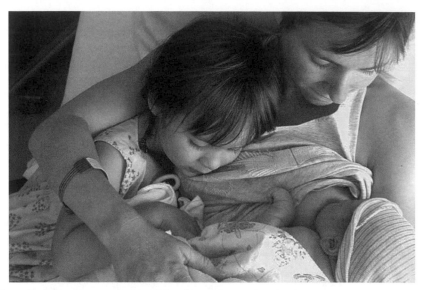

Breastfeeding gives you a free hand for older siblings and is also the best, most natural way to teach breastfeeding norms to the next generation. (©2005 Marilyn Nolt, used with permission)

common breastfeeding challenges. We wish we had a nickel for every new mother with nipple trauma who started their conversation with: "The nurses in the hospital told me my latch-on is fine." In most cases, adjusting the "fine" latch-on proved to be the key to eliminating the nipple pain.

Normal feeding patterns. We described in chapters 4 and 5 the normal breastfeeding patterns of healthy newborns. But for those of us more familiar with bottlefeeding, breastfeeding norms may not feel normal at all. As we explained, babies fed by bottle (no matter what is in the bottle) tend to take more at a feeding and feed fewer times per day. Bottle-fed newborns tend to feed six to eight times per day, whereas breastfeeding newborns tend to feed more like eight to twelve times per day. Because of the dynamics of the delivery system, bottlefeeding establishes an overfeeding pattern early in life. While not necessarily healthy, bottle-feeding norms may still feel normal, if that's what you're used to. As we said earlier, new parents are still encouraged by many to use feeding schedules. Although this can work for bottle-fed babies, scheduling can sometimes lead to breastfeeding problems such as milk supply issues and slow weight gain, which we discussed in detail in chapter 6.

Rigid feeding schedules can also lead to other breastfeeding problems. We know a lactation consultant who made a home visit to a mother just discharged from the hospital whose baby was not latching on. When she arrived, the baby was sound asleep. While filling out the paperwork, the baby started to stir. The lactation consultant said, "Why don't we come back to the paperwork later and work with the baby now. She acts as if she's ready to feed." The mother looked at the clock and said, "No. It's not time to breastfeed yet." The mother explained that she had been told at the hospital to breastfeed every three hours. She took these instructions literally and had been ignoring her baby's cues and cries, picking her up and trying to breastfeed on the dot of the third hour. At every "feeding time" the baby was either sound asleep or screaming so hard that the mother couldn't calm her to feed. The solution to her problem was very simple. As soon as she began breastfeeding when her baby showed early feeding cues (rooting, hand to mouth), breastfeeding went smoothly.

Few mothers approach breastfeeding as literally and rigidly as this mother, but her story is instructive. Bottlefeeding by the clock can work because a reluctant feeder can sometimes be "forced" to feed by pushing the firm bottle nipple into the back of baby's mouth, which triggers active sucking. But a baby who is not ready to breastfeed cannot be forced to. The baby must be willing and ready to draw the soft breast back to the comfort zone. Like a dance, breastfeeding only works if both people cooperate. Breastfeeding may be nature's first lesson in healthy human interactions.

COMMERCIAL PRESSURES

Another cultural force that undermines breastfeeding is commercial pressures. Formula is a billion-dollar industry, and like any business, it works hard to keep and increase its market share. Unfortunately, as its market share rises, breastfeeding decreases and the health of mothers and babies suffers. Many note the parallels between the tobacco industry and the formula industry, as both promote products that have proven ill effects on public health. And both the movements to stop smoking and to encourage breastfeeding require cultural change and public education in order to accomplish their goals.

Formula Marketing Aimed at Parents

Amazing as it may seem to those of us in the U.S., prior to 1991 there were no magazine ads or television commercials for infant formula in this country. The only advertising for formula was print ads appearing in medical journals that were directed at doctors. However, since formula advertising directed at parents began, a whole new challenge to breastfeeding came into being.

Earlier in this chapter, we mentioned the WHO Code, which was created to stop the marketing of infant formula to the general public. This was needed because of the many deaths resulting from unethical formula marketing practices in developing nations. But the WHO Code was not meant only for developing nations. From a public-health perspective, it makes sense to eliminate direct marketing of formula to consumers everywhere.

Although the U.S. chose not to adopt the WHO Code, for many years the formula companies did not advertise directly to parents. However, in 1991, Gerber opened the floodgates with its direct marketing campaign to consumers. Now all major formula manufacturers devote some of their considerable budgets to print and television ads for parents. In the U.S., not only are pregnant women bombarded with these formula ads, it is the rare family that does not receive coupons by mail for discounts on infant formula, cases of formula delivered directly to their door, and formula marketing bags given "free" at hospitals when they give birth. (Hospitals—supposedly promoters of public health—are rewarded financially for their role as formula endorsers and marketers.)

Most people firmly believe (despite much research to the contrary) that they are not influenced by marketing. But there is no doubt that commercial pressures have done much to normalize the use of infant formula and thereby undermine breastfeeding. In the U.S. today, it is the rare baby who does not receive at least some infant formula.

TAPPING INTO NEW PARENT ANXIETY

The following is just one example of how vulnerable new parents are targeted by formula companies to the detriment of breastfeeding.

The right formula. In 2003 at a conference for lactation professionals, Virginia Tech English professor Bernice Hausman provided a fascinating analysis of formula marketing strategies. During her fifth month of pregnancy, Hausman began receiving formula marketing materials. In the mailing that arrived just before her baby was due, along with formula coupons, she received a chart with the following headings:

My baby has . . .	Which could mean . . .	Type of formula
Problems with gas	Baby reacts to lactose	Enfamil Lactose-Free

Along with "problems with gas," other conditions in the "My baby has . . ." column included "restless sleep," "fussy times," and even "absence of a regular schedule." The second column interpreted the baby's behavior, and the third column listed which of the "Enfamil Family of Formulas" provided a solution to the baby's "problem." Of course, human milk or breastfeeding were mentioned nowhere on the chart.

This approach feeds into new parents' normal insecurities in order to sell formula. Absence of a regular schedule, fussy periods, restless sleep, and gas are all normal aspects of infancy. If formula companies successfully convince new parents that these are problems in need of a solution, they are halfway down the slippery slope to solving their problem with "the right formula." (Of course, if someone was paid to market breastfeeding using this strategy, a similar chart would include problems we know to be related to formula use, such as constipation, allergy, illness, and digestive problems, with breastfeeding listed as the solution for them all.)

These formula marketing materials also feed into the expectations created by scientific mothering, such as new parents' desire for their babies to sleep well, feed at predictable intervals, and never act fussy. They also feed into the cultural expectation many new parents have that in order to meet their baby's needs they must buy a wide variety of consumer products. As Hausman noted: "Problems are addressed through the purchase of goods. . . . Thus one goal of formula promotion materials is to identify baby behavior as problems that can be solved through a specific, informed purchase."

BREASTFEEDING AND THE MEDICAL COMMUNITY

Although some progress has been made in recent years, some of the greatest obstacles to normal breastfeeding after birth come from what appears on the face of it to be an unlikely source: the medical community. These obstacles are due in part to the inertia of institutions ("we've always done it this way") after generations of formula feeding, but commercial pressures also play a role here.

A Bottle-Feeding Mentality

Like many in the U.S., medical professions today, by and large, tend to have a "bottle-feeding mentality" because of their greater familiarity with formula feeding. The U.S. medical community is so well educated about formula and so poorly educated about breastfeeding that they often unknowingly undermine the latter.

THEY GO WITH WHAT THEY KNOW

Despite their sincere desire to help, medical providers tend to go with the familiar. The formula industry makes sure that doctors and nurses learn about formula feeding both during medical school and after. As part of their marketing efforts, the industry sponsors meals with free educational seminars and even perks such as cruises. This training also leaves health professionals with the (desired) impression that giving nonhuman milks is normal or at the very least benign. Doctors we know have also received unlimited supplies of free formula for their own babies because formula company representatives know that these doctors can be very influential in encouraging their patients to also use formula.

Because they are well-trained in bottlefeeding, when doctors and nurses are unsure about how to help a new mother make breastfeeding work, they often suggest switching to or supplementing with formula rather than referring a mother to a specialist, as they would with most other health issues. Many health professionals fed their own children formula, which makes it hard for them to accept emotionally the importance of breastfeeding.

Those doctors and nurses who do know about breastfeeding only learn about it if they happen to have a special interest in it. Then they must pursue their learning on their own and at their own expense. Another way some health providers learn about breastfeeding is if they or their spouse breastfeed. A major overhaul is desperately needed in breastfeeding education for doctors and nurses.

THE OVERUSE OF FORMULA

An outgrowth of this bottle-feeding mentality is the gross overuse of formula. Please don't misunderstand us here. Formula can a blessing in the rare cases in which it is truly needed. This need is the greatest in the U.S. and in parts of the world where donor human milk is only available on a limited basis for babies with serious health problems. In some parts of the world, like Scandanavia, babies whose mothers' milk is unavailable are routinely fed donor human milk from milk banks, avoiding the negative health outcomes of nonhuman milks.

Formula advocates. If you have not yet given birth and you prefer your baby not be given formula, be prepared. Depending upon the institution, formula supplementation may not only be routine, it may also be very difficult to prevent. As one lactation consultant writes:

> In a survey I conducted in Utah, 25 percent of the nurses felt formula was so important to a baby's well-being that they would give formula even if the physician or mother specifically said not to.
>
> By experience I learned that there are some staff members who feel so sorry for the breastfed babies (who seem to get fed so little compared to formula-fed babies) that they will take any opportunity to feed them, truly feeling that they are looking out for the babies' welfare better than the misguided mothers and doctors who want the baby

to be exclusively breastfed. They can be strengthened in this belief if there is one physician who vocalizes the same beliefs, though he be only one physician of many.

—Arly Helm, MS, IBCLC (2004)

As we described in the introduction, the premature introduction of nonhuman milks can put your baby at risk for allergies and a variety of other health problems. Despite its overuse, formula is *not* benign to either breastfeeding or to your baby. It may sometimes be necessary, but most often it is given unnecessarily. In some birthing facilities, nurses know so little about normal breastfeeding that they believe new-borns' desire to feed long and often in the early days means that these babies need formula supplements. Many new mothers are undermined in their desire to exclusively breastfeed by health-care providers who tell them they don't have enough milk.

How to avoid formula exposure. If you give birth in a hospital and want to avoid exposing your baby to formula, the best way is to take advantage of "rooming-in" and keep your baby with you at all times. If that isn't possible, the next best thing is to get an order of "no supple-ments" in writing from your baby's health-care provider. If your baby's usual health-care provider is not on staff where you will be giving birth, your baby will be assigned a doctor on staff and that doctor's orders will be followed until your baby is discharged. In this case, you'll need to get a no-supplement order in writing from the doctor on staff. It isn't enough for the doctor to promise this verbally. If your baby's doctor's orders include routine supplementation, you need to go to the hospital with your exception in writing, signed by the doctor, and give copies to those caring for your baby. If you don't, your baby may be given supple-ments until the doctor says otherwise.

SUMMARY

As you can see, there are some major forces at work that can undermine breastfeeding. At one point in the not-too-distant past, breastfeeding was in danger of dying out in the U.S. Breastfeeding had no backing from major scientific organizations (that has certainly changed!) and had no international organizations working for its success. The only thing it did have was the very real health drawbacks of other methods of infant feeding.

Yet despite all the forces that have conspired against breastfeeding, breastfeeding rates are continuing to rise in the U.S., increasing an average of about 1 percent annually over the past decade. Knowing about the forces that interfere with the laws is important in neutralizing their influence. After all, knowledge is power. Understanding these dynamics can help you distinguish good advice from bad advice and good breastfeeding information from questionable breastfeeding information. This knowledge gives you a better perspective from which to make important decisions for you, for your baby, and for your whole family.

PART II

Applying the Laws

CHAPTER 9

Daily Life with Your Breastfeeding Baby

Having a baby changes every aspect of your life. But you probably already know that! You may sometimes long for your former life B.C.— before children. Your B.C. days may be over, but you can embrace a new normal that includes life with your baby. As a breastfeeding woman, you can still be a part of the wider world. This chapter will help you to make this transition.

REENTERING THE WORLD WITH YOUR BREASTFEEDING BABY

Reentering the world means being out and about with your baby. Breastfeeding can simplify this. There may also be times when you need to be away from your baby. We offer some suggestions on how you can do both.

Out with Baby

As a new mother, you may wonder about how best to handle feedings when you and your baby venture out of the house. No one thinks twice about giving a baby a bottle in public. Yet many women worry about offending others by breastfeeding. What are some of your options when breastfeeding away from home?

YOU CAN BREASTFEED ANYWHERE

If you feel nervous about breastfeeding in public, learning how to feed your baby discreetly can help. Some mothers drape a blanket over their shoulder to cover the baby. Others wrap the baby in the blanket and pull the corner up over their breast. This allows you to see your baby, and it doesn't cover the baby's head and face, which bothers some babies.

Discreet breastfeeding is easier if you wear a two-piece outfit. You can lift your top from the bottom, with your baby's body covering any exposed skin. Jackets, cardigan sweaters, and over-blouses also provide extra coverage. There are also special breastfeeding fashions with openings and panels to make discreet nursing even easier. (See our Web site for further information). Many women have gained confidence by practicing in front of a mirror or having your partner take a look.

Baby slings can also be helpful. Many mothers find nursing a baby in a sling the height of ease and modesty because they either use the tail of the sling as a cover-up or pull up the extra fabric of the sling to cover the baby. This allows them to breastfeed while walking around public places with no one the wiser.

YOU CAN FIND A PRIVATE PLACE

Even mothers who are usually comfortable breastfeeding in public may sometimes prefer more privacy. Some shopping centers and other public arenas offer special areas for breastfeeding moms. Other options include changing rooms, lounges, or benches in a quiet part of the mall. To make breastfeeding less obvious in a restaurant, you may choose to sit at a table in the back of the restaurant, with your back toward the front. A restroom is probably the least desirable place to breastfeed (it's not a great place for anyone to eat, especially a baby). But it can be an option, if needed.

Family gatherings may also present a challenge, especially if you're the first one in your family to breastfeed. Depending on those in attendance, you may choose to breastfeed in another room—or not. Some mothers will abide by others' preferences in someone else's home, but not when in their own homes. With more exposure (no pun intended!), many families gain a greater comfort level with breastfeeding.

MANY U.S. STATES HAVE BREASTFEEDING LAWS

A number of U.S. states have passed laws protecting a woman's right to breastfeed in public. These laws came about because some women were harassed for breastfeeding in restaurants, shopping malls, and even doctors' offices. These laws do not require discreet breast-feeding, as they rightly assume that there's nothing indecent about feeding your baby. (It's the normal way for a baby to eat!) But these laws were necessary because sometimes even discreetly breastfeeding mothers were hassled or asked to leave when someone discovered that they were breastfeeding. To see if your state has such a law, refer to our Web site for a listing.

AWAY FROM YOUR BABY

In chapter 2, we explained why a mother's body is a baby's natural habi-tat, and that separation is physically stressful for babies. In chapter 5, we described different types of mammalian feeding patterns and concluded that humans are "carry mammals," which require constant carrying and feeding. Understanding human biology gives you a great perspective on your baby. It helps you appreciate why she gets so upset when you put her down and why skin-to-skin contact with you gives her such pleasure.

Sorting Out Your Feelings

But understanding it and living it may be an entirely different matter. Perhaps you have decided to do whatever it takes to never miss a breastfeeding. Maybe you wish you could live your life that way, but practicalities interfere. It could be that you consider feeding only directly from the breast interesting to think about, but have no desire to be with your baby 24/7. Whatever your situation or your preference, you can still make breastfeeding work.

How to Handle Times Apart

When considering time you and your baby are apart, there are a number of ways to handle breastfeeding.

Time your outings so that you don't miss feedings. If your baby is somewhat regular in her breastfeeding patterns, you may be able to slip out between feedings without having to leave any milk behind.

Make arrangements to have your baby brought to you at feeding times. Try to be creative when thinking of ways to get your baby to you to feed. You may have more latitude than you think. While not every setting is appropriate for a baby, it may be possible to have someone bring the baby to you when it's time to breastfeed.

Follow your heart. This is ultimately your decision. If you do not want to be away from your baby, don't let others pressure you to. There's nothing that says being away is necessary for everyone. And if you need or want to be away, that's your decision, too.

This too shall pass. It's so easy to lose perspective during the intense early months when you're adjusting to motherhood. Some women worry that this stage of intense mothering will last forever. As two experienced mothers, we can tell you that this stage actually goes by pretty quickly. When you allow yourself to relish to its fullest the closeness and intimacy you can have with your baby, you gain a depth and a richness in your life that wasn't there before you had children. Think of this intense time as an opportunity for personal growth. Instead of trying to hurry this phase along or believe the cultural messages that you "need" to get away from your baby, try as much as possible to relax and enjoy this time together.

In almost every situation, it's still possible to breastfeed. Even mothers who need to be away from their babies for extended periods (such as women who work full-time and travel) still maintain their milk supplies when they are away and breastfeed when they are with their babies.

Leave your milk for your baby. If you will be away at a feeding time, you can leave some expressed milk for your baby. If you're gone longer than your baby's longest sleep stretch or your breasts start to feel full, you'll also need to pump your breasts while you are gone to keep up your milk supply and to prevent mastitis.

Leave formula for your baby. If you prefer not to leave your milk, or for some reason cannot, there is always the option of giving formula while you're away. As we've said throughout, some breastfeeding is always better than none.

BOTTLE FEEDING

If your baby is older than one month of age and you need to be away, chances are that your caregiver will feed your baby with a bottle (see chapter 11 for alternatives for babies younger than one month of age). Bottles are the most common alternative to the breast in developed countries. Bottles are familiar. They are readily available and inexpensive. But bottles are not without controversy. One concern is that babies may come to prefer bottles and then have difficulty going back to the breast, especially if bottles are given during the first month. Some people call this "nipple confusion." For some babies, this can be a legitimate concern. However, most babies go to the breast just fine even when they've had bottles. Unfortunately, babies are not born with labels to know which are easily confused and which ones are not. If you're planning to use bottles, here are some strategies that are less likely to compromise breastfeeding.

Wait until your baby's about three to four weeks old. Despite what many people say, studies show it doesn't really seem to matter how late you start bottle feeding. Approximately 70 percent of babies take a bottle easily whether you start at one month, two months, or even three to six months. Another 26 percent of babies require some patience and persistence to accept a bottle. And a few babies (about 4 percent) refuse a bottle no matter what (Kearney and Cronenwett 1991). But keep in mind that babies also can be fed with a cup, spoon, or dropper (see chapter 11).

Have someone else give the bottle. Your baby may not be willing to take a bottle from you because she's smart enough to know she could be nursing instead. She may not take a bottle if you are even in the building. Have the caregiver try giving a bottle for the first time when baby is not too hungry. If the baby won't take the bottle in the nursing position, try other positions. A good long-term strategy for a baby receiving regular bottles is to confine bottle feeding to the caregiver and breastfeeding to mom.

Pick a bottle your baby likes. The best bottle is the type your baby likes. Start by buying several types of bottles and nipples and see how your baby responds to them. Some recommended brands include Avent and Johnson's Healthflow.

Employment Outside the Home

The question of whether to work outside the home is one that many mothers wrestle with. Fortunately, you can continue breastfeeding even if you and your baby are regularly apart. In this case, to meet your breastfeeding goals, it helps to plan ahead.

BEFORE GOING BACK TO WORK

Before you head back to work, advance planning can help make this transition as smooth as possible.

Decide on your breastfeeding goals. Breastfeeding doesn't have to be all or nothing. Your choices include:

- maintaining a full milk supply and supplying only mother's milk for the feedings you and your baby are apart;

- supplying as much mother's milk as is convenient, using formula as needed;

- supplementing with formula while away; breastfeeding when together.

Consider your work options. The number of hours you work and the type of work you do can affect breastfeeding. Will you work full-time or part-time? How old will baby be when you return to work? Waiting until your baby is at least three months old can improve your chances of keeping up your milk supply long-term. Can you work from home? Are there job-sharing options? Flex-time? Can you take your baby to work? Can baby be brought to you at work for feedings? See our Web site (www.Breast feedingMadeSimple.com) for more employment options.

Find a breastfeeding-friendly caregiver. Look for a caregiver supportive of breastfeeding. Finding one close to work (rather than close to home) might allow you to breastfeed baby at breaks by either going to your baby or having your baby brought to you. If you breastfeed at the caregiver's before leaving for work, it also cuts down on your time apart, decreasing the amount of milk needed while you're away.

Build your supply of expressed milk. Allow at least three to four weeks before starting back to work to get practiced with your method of milk expression and to start storing milk. Keep in mind that once at work, the milk you express one day can be left for the next day. If you express milk just once a day for three weeks, you'll have enough milk for your first day back to work and a good reserve.

MAKE ARRANGEMENTS AT WORK

Before you return to work, talk with your employer about what help you will need to continue to breastfeed. Let your company know that your continuing to breastfeed benefits them. When companies support breastfeeding, women return to work more quickly, use fewer health-care dollars, take fewer sick days, and report greater job satisfaction, resulting in reduced staff turnover. (See our Web site for information you can share with your employer.) Here is some of what you will need in your workplace.

Find a place to express. You will need a place to express your milk where you can relax and have some privacy. Ask if you can use a private office, conference room, storage room, or lounge. A bathroom is not ideal because it isn't sanitary. But if it's your only option, you can make it work. If you're using a breast pump and an electrical outlet is not available, some breast pumps can be powered by batteries, battery packs, or even car adapters.

Allow twenty minutes per session. If you are using a double pump, allow ten to fifteen minutes per pumping session and five minutes for clean-up. *If you plan to keep up a full milk supply and provide your baby exclusively with your milk, divide the number of hours away from baby, including travel time, by three* (for example, nine hours away means three pumpings). Depending on their breast storage capacity (see chapter 6), some mothers can provide enough milk with fewer pumping sessions.

Have a place to store milk. You can store your milk at room temperature for up to four to six hours. However, if you are away for longer than this, you'll need to cool your milk. Cooling choices include a separate cooler compartment in your pump case, separate cooler bag, or refrigerator. Fresh and cooled batches of milk can be combined (though fresh milk must be cooled before being added to frozen milk). Human milk is *not* a biohazard, and no unusual precautions are needed.

CHOOSING A METHOD OF EXPRESSION

If you are planning to supply your milk while you're away, another decision you'll need to make is how to express your milk. For more information, see the later section "Expressing and Storing Milk."

If you choose to use a breast pump, below are our suggestions for pumps best suited for full- and part-time work. The type of pump most likely to meet your needs will depend upon the amount of time you're away from your baby.

Away from baby full-time. If your goal is to keep up your milk supply and you'll be away from baby for feedings thirty to forty-plus hours per week, your choices include Ameda or Medela rental pumps. Or you may purchase the Ameda Purely Yours or one of the Medela Pump In Styles. These pumps provide you with similar stimulation as a baby actively nursing (forty to sixty suction-and-release cycles per minute). Most women find that using a pump that is limited to fewer cycles leads to a gradually decreasing supply. When pricing pumps, keep in mind that formula costs between $100 to $250 U.S. per month. A good pump is an investment that pays back many times over.

Away from baby part-time. If you'll be working part-time, you'll miss fewer feedings and have more options in terms of pumps. The above pumps will work well, but if you plan to pump less often than once a day, consider pumps that provide fewer cycles per minute. If your number of work hours is very limited, you may even do well with a good manual pump.

ONCE YOU'RE BACK AT WORK

To keep up your milk supply over the long-term, don't forget Law 6: "More milk out equals more milk made."

Plan to breastfeed as much as possible. A good goal is to keep the total number of breast drainings (breastfeedings plus pumpings) per twenty-four hours the same as before you started work. Consider breast-feeding your baby twice in the morning: once when you wake up, and again right before you leave her. Plan to breastfeed as soon as you see baby after work. If your baby seems hungry right before you arrive, suggest the caregiver give as little milk as possible until you get there. If your baby starts sleeping longer at night and overall number of breast drainings decrease, think about when you can fit in more at other times.

Learn how to encourage milk flow. Work can sometimes be stressful, and stress can inhibit milk release and slow milk flow. If you sit down to

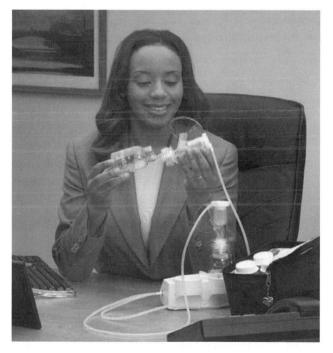

The Ameda Purely Yours breast pump is a good choice for women who work full-time and plan to pump at work. (©2005 Hollister, Inc, used with permission of Hollister, Inc., Libertyville, IL)

pump and the milk is not flowing, see the section "Expressing to Store Milk" for tips.

Know how to stop leaks. Not all women leak. If you do, use nursing pads or LilyPadz, a silicone product that applies gentle pressure to your nipples to stop milk flow (see our Resources section). You can also wear patterned blouses instead of solids to camouflage, or have a cardigan sweater or jacket handy as a cover up. Regular pumping will minimize leaking, but if you feel a leak starting, you can stop the flow by discreetly applying pressure to the nipples with your forearms.

Increase your milk supply. If your milk supply dips, you should be able to increase it, especially if you act on it right away. *Don't wait.* Read the section on increasing your milk supply in chapter 10.

LIFESTYLE ISSUES

Breastfeeding evolved as a normal part of life. That means there aren't a long list of rules you must follow to make it work; just the basic principles we described in part 1. Here is more information related to commonly asked questions.

Food, Drink, and Other Consumables

Contrary to popular belief, there are no foods that you should eat or avoid while you're breastfeeding. You don't have to drink milk, for example, to make milk.

EVERYTHING IN MODERATION

Your body has the amazing ability to make milk out of anything you eat—pizza, roast beef, or garbanzo beans. Similarly, there are no foods you must avoid. You can eat chocolate, spicy foods, onions, garlic, broccoli, cabbage. The key is: *everything in moderation*. The cuisines of many countries are spicy and flavorful (for instance, Thailand and Mexico). Mothers in these countries eat spicy foods while breastfeeding with no ill effects on their babies. Enjoy!

Eat to hunger. Extra calories do not seem to be as important as was once believed. Just eat to satisfy your hunger. The fat stores you built up during pregnancy provide much of the fuel needed to establish milk production. Research also indicates that your metabolism may be more efficient while nursing than at other times, reducing your need for extra calories (Illingsworth et al. 1986). If you are more active, you will need more calories—but you will also feel hungrier. You can diet while breastfeeding. In fact, this may be a very good time, as formula-feeding mothers tend to lose weight more slowly than those who breastfeed. But it's best to go slowly and lose weight gradually. Any diet plan should include at least 1800 calories a day.

Sometimes mothers wonder whether something they've eaten is affecting their babies. If you are concerned, keep in mind that almost all babies have fussy periods. Your baby's fussiness is probably unrelated to your diet. If you suspect a food is affecting her, try eliminating the food from your diet. It may take a couple of weeks for you to notice a difference. For example, cow's milk and dairy, the most common cause of problems, takes two weeks or so to clear. After you've eliminated it, then try reintroducing it. The most likely culprits are protein foods such as dairy, soy, egg white, peanuts, meat, and fish. Only diet elimination trials will tell you for sure.

Drink to thirst. How much fluid should you drink while breastfeeding? "Drink to thirst" is the simple guideline. Despite the common belief to the contrary, research has not yet found a connection between a mother's fluid intake and her milk supply. If your urine is dark yellow, you need more fluids. To make it easy to get a drink when thirsty, keep a container of water or juice at your usual nursing spot.

CAFFEINE, ALCOHOL, AND CIGARETTES

When it comes to caffeine, alcohol, and cigarettes, again, moderation is important.

Caffeine. You may have abstained from caffeine during pregnancy, but there's no need to do so while breastfeeding. Research indicates that a mother can consume up to five cups of coffee before her breastfeeding baby is affected (Nehlig and Debry 1994). One or two cups of coffee or other caffeinated drinks per day will not cause a problem for most breastfeeding mothers and babies.

Alcohol. An occasional beer or glass of wine is also acceptable while breastfeeding. Moderate to heavy drinking would put a baby at risk. But occasional exposure to alcohol through the milk has not been found to be harmful. If you feel strongly that you don't want your baby exposed to any alcohol, you can simply allow time for it to clear from your system. The alcohol from one glass of beer or wine is out of the milk of a 120 lb. woman within two to three hours, for example (Schulte 1995). You don't need to pump your milk for the alcohol to pass out of it— alcohol leaves your milk automatically as blood alcohol levels decrease. If a breastfeeding mother has a stronger drink or more than one glass of beer or wine, it would take much longer for her milk to be free of alcohol.

Smoking. If you smoke, it is still better for you to breastfeed your baby. The benefits of human milk far outweigh any risk associated with nicotine exposure. Don't smoke around your baby or let others do so, as this can increase the risk of SIDS. And try to cut down on the number of cigarettes you smoke in a day. The fewer cigarettes you smoke, the better it is for you and your baby.

Exercise and Personal Grooming

There are many benefits to exercising after you have a baby. It reduces stress and depression, makes you feel better, and aids in weight loss. Similarly, being able to engage in grooming routines will help you feel better and bring a renewed sense of normalcy to your life. Below are further details.

YOU CAN EXERCISE

Sometimes mothers wonder whether it's okay to exercise while breastfeeding. The short answer is yes. One early study raised a concern about whether enough of a substance called lactic acid accumulated in a woman's milk during exercise to cause babies to refuse the breast. Subsequent studies have found this not to be an issue (see Mohrbacher and Stock 2003 for a review of this research).

Breastfeeding mothers do *not* need to restrict their exercise. You can exercise alone or find an exercise that you and your baby can do together: mom and baby exercise class, walking with the baby in a stroller or carrier, or running with a jogging stroller.

PERMS, HAIR DYES, TANNING BEDS, AND PIERCINGS

Hair dye and permanents are also okay for breastfeeding mothers. There is no evidence that hair-care products get into a mother's milk. Similarly, tanning beds do not have any impact on your milk. Nor does nipple piercing. Women with pierced nipples can still breastfeed their babies.

EXPRESSING AND STORING MILK

Expressing milk refers to removing it from your breasts, either manually or with a breast pump. Not all breastfeeding mothers need to express their milk. But for most women who breastfeed for any length of time, knowing how to express milk is a useful skill.

Milk Expression Basics

There are many reasons women express their milk. The following are the most common.

To stay comfortable. This is most likely to happen during the first week or so after birth, when a mother's breasts may feel full even after her baby breastfeeds. This may also be useful during weaning.

To provide milk for feedings and/or stimulate milk supply. These may be important when:

- a mother and her baby are separated at feeding times;

- the baby is unable or unwilling to breastfeed;

- the baby is not breastfeeding effectively;

- a mother wants a partner or the baby's siblings to feed the baby or prefers to feed her milk by bottle in some situations;

- a mother want to increase her milk supply by draining her breasts more often or more fully.

METHODS OF MILK EXPRESSION

In many parts of the world, women express their milk by hand. However, in the U.S., women most commonly express milk with a breast pump. If you use a pump, you may find the following tips helpful.

Give yourself time to practice. If you are pumping, know that it takes time to get accustomed to a breast pump and become proficient in its use. Even with an ample milk supply, some mothers find it difficult to express their milk, especially at first and even with a good pump. If you need to express your milk on a regular basis, be sure to give yourself enough time to learn to use your pump and to become used to its feel.

Find the right fit. The better pump companies (Hollister and Medela) offer flanges with different-sized nipple tunnels. If your nipples are rubbing uncomfortably along the sides of the pump nipple tunnel or you're not getting good results, try a larger size.

EXPRESSING TO STORE MILK

If you're pumping to store milk, the following basics may be of help.

Try pumping in the morning. Most women get more milk in the morning than later in the day. A good time to pump is usually thirty to sixty minutes after a nursing and at least an hour before a breastfeeding. The worst time is right before breastfeeding.

Enhance your milk release. Removing milk with a pump is not like sucking liquid through a straw. With a straw, the stronger you suck, the more liquid you get. With the breast, strength of suction has little to do with effective pumping (Mitoulas et al. 2002). The key to expressing milk is triggering the letdown, or milk release (for more information, see chapter 2).

During milk release, the breast actively moves the milk toward the nipple, where the baby or pump can access it. Muscles within the breast squeeze to push the milk out and the ducts widen. Some mothers feel this as a tingling sensation in their breasts; others feel nothing. A milk release can be triggered by a certain touch at the breast, hearing another mother's baby cry, or even by thinking about your baby. Feelings of tension, anger, or frustration can block it. Without a milk release, a mother will only express the small amount of milk pooled around the nipple. So triggering milk release is vital to successful pumping.

During breastfeeding, most mothers have several milk releases without even knowing it (Ramsay et al. 2004). When your baby is at the breast, all the familiar physical cues (softness, warmth) and your loving emotions release the hormones that trigger milk release.

When a mother puts a pump to her breasts, though, these normal baby cues are missing. For this reason, some mothers need a little extra help at first in triggering milk releases as they adjust to the new feel of the pump. This can also happen when a mother switches from one pump to another (even one hospital-grade pump to another), because the feel of the pump is different.

If you need some help releasing your milk to the pump, experiment with the following suggestions, and see which work for you. You may only need to use one or two for a short time until the feel of the pump becomes familiar.

- *Feelings:* Close your eyes, relax, and imagine your baby is breastfeeding. Breathe slowly and deeply and think about how much you love your baby.

- *Sight:* Look at your baby or, if away from your baby, look at her photo.

- *Hearing:* Listen to a tape recording of your baby cooing or crying. If you're away, call your baby's caregiver and check on her. Call someone you love to relax and distract you.

- *Smell:* Smell an item of your baby's clothing or her blanket.

- *Touch:* Apply warm compresses or gently massage your breasts.

- *Taste:* Sip a favorite warm drink to relax you.

The bottom line is: more milk releases mean more milk expressed.

How much milk to expect per pumping. If you are pumping between regular feedings and exclusively breastfeeding (using no formula and your baby is gaining well), expect to pump about half a feeding. If you are pumping at feeding time for a missed feeding, expect a full feeding. (Feeding amount will vary depending on your baby's age. See next section.)

DECIDING HOW MUCH MILK TO LEAVE FOR YOUR BABY

To help you determine how much milk to leave for feedings, use the following calculation. Babies usually take about 2.5 ounces (75 ml) of milk per pound of body weight in a twenty-four-hour period, up to a total of 30 to 35 ounces (890 to 1035 ml) per day. For example, a twelve-pound (5.4 kg) baby will take a total of about 30 ounces (890 ml) of milk in a twenty-four-hour period, which equals about 4 ounces (120 ml) per feeding for eight feedings.

HANDLING AND STORING HUMAN MILK

You will no doubt notice that milk storage guidelines differ from book to book, and it may help you to know why. Although your milk will not spoil before the times listed below, the longer it is stored, the more nutritional value is lost. That's why some suggest shorter guidelines. It is always good to use your milk as quickly as you can after expressing it. But if you should find some stored milk in the back of your refrigerator that has been sitting there for seven days, one thing is for sure—it will still be much better for your baby than formula, which doesn't provide any illness prevention. In fact, it's those antibodies—the living parts of your milk—that kill bacteria in your milk, making it hardier than formula. When in doubt, smell or taste your milk. Spoiled milk will smell spoiled.

Storage Time for Human Milk
(for full-term, healthy babies)

Freshly expressed human milk

Freezer	Refrigerator	Room temperature (<79°F; 25°C)
3–4 months in a refrigerator/freezer *(in sealed container)*	8 days (mature milk)	12–24 hours (colostrum—to day 5) 4-6 hours (mature milk)
6–12 months in a deep freeze (0°F; -19°C or lower)		

Freshly expressed milk also can be kept at <60°F (15°C) for up to 24 hours (e.g., in a bag with cooling elements).

Previously frozen human milk (*best thawed under warm running water*)

Do not refreeze	24 hours	1 hour

There is no research indicating whether freshly expressed, leftover human milk that has been warmed and given should be discarded or saved. The current guidelines from La Leche League International state that you can use this milk at the next feeding only.

These guidelines mean you can store freshly expressed milk at room temperature for four to six hours, then move it to the refrigerator for eight days, and then still freeze it. Fresh cooled milk can be added to frozen milk as long as the amount of fresh milk is not greater than the amount of milk already frozen.

You can store your milk in any clean, sealed container, but you'll want to avoid using thin bottle liners, which can split when frozen. Store your milk in amounts no larger than you think your baby will take at one feeding. This will minimize waste and make it faster for you to warm it for a feeding. Having smaller amounts also allows you to give your baby more if she wants it. When warming milk, keep heat to a minimum, as high heat kills antibodies in the milk that keep your baby healthy. If your milk is frozen, thaw it in its container under cool then warmer running water until the milk is between room temperature and body temperature.

Before you give your milk to your baby, gently swirl the container to mix the layers that have separated. (It is not homogenized like cow's milk from the store.) You can combine previously expressed milk with newly expressed milk if both are within the storage guidelines. When storing a combined batch of milk, date it according to the oldest milk. (Example: If refrigerated milk expressed on March 10 is combined with milk expressed on March 14, it should be marked with a March 10 date.)

To freeze or not to freeze? If refrigerated milk will not be used within eight days, you'll need to freeze it. If you're storing milk prior to working outside the home, plan to freeze some milk for your first day back at work, as well as a reserve for off days. Once you start working, though, plan to give mostly fresh or refrigerated milk, as freezing kills some of the antibodies in the milk that keep baby healthy. But even with fewer antibodies than fresh milk, it is still a huge improvement over formula.

MEDICATIONS AND CONTRACEPTION

At some point while you're breastfeeding, you may need to take prescription or over-the-counter (OTC) medications. Most mothers do. According to Thomas Hale, R.Ph., Ph.D., author of *Medications and Mothers' Milk*, surveys indicate that between 90 to 99 percent of mothers take medications in their first week postpartum (Hale 2004).

What to Do If You Need to Take Medications

You might wonder if a medication prescribed for you could harm your breastfeeding baby. Some mothers are so fearful of this that they choose to wean their babies rather than risk exposure to the medication. This is a common reason women give for weaning their babies prematurely. However, weaning is almost always unnecessary. If you are taking medication, don't assume that your choice is between "contaminated" breast milk and "pristine" formula. According to the American Academy of Pediatrics, in the vast majority of cases, the risks of giving formula to your baby far outweigh the risks of continuing to breastfeed with a tiny bit of medication in your milk. And for most medications, your baby is only exposed to a very small amount of what you take (often less than 1 percent of your dose). There are very few medications that are not recommended for nursing mothers (Hale 2004).

Space does not permit us to list here all the medications that are compatible with breastfeeding. But there are two resources you might find helpful. The first is the American Academy of Pediatrics's publication *The Transfer of Medications and Other Chemicals into Human Milk.* This is available on our Web site for you to share with your doctor. The second resource is Thomas Hale's *Medications and Mothers' Milk* (2004). In the lactation field, this is considered the "bible" of drug use for nursing mothers. It is updated often and is relatively inexpensive. You might want to get a copy for yourself, especially if you frequently take medications. Order information is listed in our Resources section and on our Web site. You can also call your local La Leche League leader or lactation consultant and ask them to look up any medications that you have questions about. Most have a copy of *Medications and Mothers' Milk* and can answer your question.

WHEN YOUR DOCTOR TELLS YOU TO WEAN

If a health-care provider recommends weaning, chances are it isn't necessary. If your doctor is relying on the *Physicians' Desk Reference* (PDR), you should know that the information about breastfeeding is often inaccurate. Drug manufacturers compile the PDR, and they are often more concerned about possible legal action (hence, the caution about advising breastfeeding moms not to use many medications) than they are about giving unbiased information on drugs and breastfeeding.

In contrast, *Medications and Mothers' Milk* looks specifically at the characteristics of the medication, how your body processes it, and how much is detectable in infants whose mothers have taken it. In most cases, if there is any medication detectable in the infant's blood, it is far below what would be considered a "clinical" dose (or a dose big enough to have any impact). Sharing this information with your baby's doctor is often enough to reassure them that the medication is compatible with breastfeeding. It's always in your best interest to be open with your health-care provider about medications that you're taking (including OTC, herbal, and prescription medications), and to tell them that you are breastfeeding when any drugs are prescribed for you. Also, be aware of the possibility that something you are taking may interact with something that your baby is taking. The safest course is to tell your health-care provider about everything that both you and your baby are taking.

SOME GENERAL GUIDELINES ON MEDICATION USE

Even though most medications are compatible with breastfeeding, you want to be sensible in their use. Here are some of Thomas Hale's (2004) general guidelines.

- *The smallest dose is best.* It's in your and your baby's best interest to use the smallest therapeutic dose that will help you. Take only the amount prescribed.

- *Your baby's age, weight, and the number of times she breastfeeds all make a difference.* Babies who are older, heavier, or who eat other foods (meaning that they breastfeed less) have less exposure to medications than babies who are premature, ill, small, or exclusively breastfeeding. However, even in the case of small or young babies, the exposure to medication is almost always less risky than weaning.

- *Drugs given to babies are usually okay for mothers to take.* If a medication is normally prescribed for infants to take (for example, amoxicillin), then it is generally appropriate for breastfeeding mothers to take. However, don't assume that a drug you took while pregnant is automatically fine for you to take while breastfeeding. Your body processes medications differently during pregnancy than after your baby is born. It's always good to double-check.

HERBAL MEDICATIONS

In the past decade, herbal medications have received a huge surge in interest. There are a number of advantages of herbs over traditional pharmaceutical medications, such as lower costs (especially for someone without prescription coverage), easier access, and fewer side effects. All of these factors are important and may be why you are considering taking herbs. Unfortunately, people often avoid telling their health-care providers that they are taking herbs for fear that their providers will judge them. We can understand why this happens, but it is a dangerous practice in general, and particularly now that you are breastfeeding. We need to caution you that just because something is "natural" doesn't mean you should be careless in its use. *Herbs are drugs,* just like their pharmacologic counterparts. You should only take them if you have a specific need. Your safest course is to work with a licensed herbalist or other health-care provider who is knowledgeable about herbs.

There are three good sources of information on the compatibility of herbs with breastfeeding: *Nursing Mother's Herbal* by Sheila Humphrey (2003), *The German Commission E Monographs* (Blumenthal et al. 1998), and *Medications and Mothers' Milk* by Thomas Hale. For information on where to find them, see our References section or our Web site.

Contraception

Your choice of contraception may have an impact on breastfeeding, but most methods do not. Here is a brief summary of what you need to know.

CONTRACEPTION WITH NO EFFECT ON BREASTFEEDING

If you live in an industrialized country, you may be surprised to learn that breastfeeding itself is contraceptive—if breastfeeding meets certain criteria.

Lactation as contraception. Breastfeeding as contraception (called the Lactation Amenorrhea Method or LAM) is most effective if a mother's periods have not returned and if the baby is:

- not receiving other liquids or solids;

- not going longer than four hours between breastfeedings during the day and six hours at night;

- younger than six months old.

If a mother's periods have returned, she is supplementing, or going longer between feedings, her risk of pregnancy is increased. This explains why we all know of women who have gotten pregnant while breastfeeding. On the other hand, if a woman is exclusively breastfeeding, meaning that the baby receives no other liquids or solids, and she meets the other criteria, the contraceptive effect of breastfeeding is around 98 percent.

Natural Family Planning. Another nonhormonal form of birth control is Natural Family Planning (NFP). NFP teaches women to observe their body signs, such as changes in temperature, cervical mucus, and in the opening of the cervix to determine times when she is fertile. She can then plan the timing of intercourse appropriately. Training is necessary for women to learn their fertility signals.

Barrier methods. Barrier methods, such as condoms, diaphragms, contraceptive sponges, or cervical caps are also effective, relatively inexpensive, and have no impact on breastfeeding. If spermicides are used, these are considered compatible with breastfeeding (Mohrbacher and Stock 2003).

Nonhormonal IUDs. Nonhormonal intrauterine devices (IUDs) are another possible method with no impact on breastfeeding. It is best if you have it inserted within two to four days after birth, or after six weeks postpartum.

Sterilization. Tubal ligation is another method of contraception with no impact on breastfeeding. However, if you choose to have surgery immediately after birth, you will be separated from your baby, which will affect your ability to breastfeed frequently in the early days. You might consider delaying this procedure until breastfeeding is well established. A hysterectomy (full or partial, even with removal of the ovaries) will not affect breastfeeding.

HORMONAL METHODS OF CONTRACEPTION

Because the artificial hormones in hormonal birth control sometimes affect milk supply, they are not the first choice for breastfeeding mothers. However, hormonal methods that use progestin only are considered compatible with breastfeeding (AAP Committee on Drugs 2001). Progestin-only methods include the minipill, progestin-IUDs, progestin-releasing vaginal rings, injectable contraceptives (such as Depo-Provera), and contraceptive implants (such as Norplant). Avoid these methods until you are at least six to eight weeks postpartum (Mohrbacher and Stock 2003).

Hormonal contraceptives with estrogen are not your best choice because estrogen can lower your milk supply—in some cases, dramatically. If you decide to use an estrogen-based contraceptive, current recommendations are that you wait until your baby is at least six months old and eating other foods.

CHAPTER 10

Common Breastfeeding Challenges

Breastfeeding is a learned skill and it can take time for it to feel natural. As you learn, you may encounter some challenges along the way. These challenges can be discouraging, but most can be overcome. Below are some suggestions for dealing with the bumps in the road you and your baby might encounter.

MOTHER-RELATED CHALLENGES

As we described in the first seven chapters, most of these challenges can be avoided by following the laws. But sometimes, even with the best intentions, life interferes and problems arise.

Engorgement

Engorgement in the early postpartum period occurs when increasing circulation, growing milk supply, and retained tissue fluid "balloon" the breast beyond its comfortable capacity, according to Jean Cotterman, RNC, IBCLC. In its extreme forms, it may feel as though your breasts are going to burst. Engorgement can make the areola firm, making a deep latch difficult, and sometimes causing the nipple to flatten. The areola must be soft enough to change shape during suckling, to let the nipple extend deep into the baby's mouth. When the breast becomes too firm, your baby may be unable to achieve this deep latch, putting you at risk for nipple pain and preventing the baby's tongue and jaws from pressing effectively on milk ducts within the breast.

WHAT YOU CAN DO

There are several things you can do to get you over this hurdle.

Drain your breasts frequently and well. Breastfeed your baby at least eight to twelve times a day. Try to breastfeed at least every hour and a half to two hours during the day and every two to three hours at night until engorgement has subsided. Make sure that your baby has a good latch and that you're in the comfort zone (see chapter 3). If your baby is not breastfeeding or breastfeeding well, use a rental pump to drain your breasts well and often. Removing milk from your breasts relieves the congestion and helps the engorgement subside more quickly.

Avoid bottles, pacifiers, or supplements. Keep your baby at the breast for all suckling. However, if your baby is not breastfeeding well, the baby obviously still needs to be fed. The best milk to use is your own given in a cup, spoon, syringe, or bottle. See chapter 11 for more on feeding methods.

Relieve pressure. When you are engorged, your baby may not be able to latch on well. If that is the case, you have a few options including reverse pressure softening, breast compression while baby breastfeeds (see the upcoming section "Sleepy Baby"), hand expression, and gentle pumping. Reverse pressure softening (RPS) a simple technique developed by Jean Cotterman, RNC, IBCLC, is a way to temporarily soften the areola (pigmented area around the nipple), making latching and milk removal easier by moving some swelling slightly backward and upward into the breast. For full instructions and line drawings, see our Web site.

Use warmth. Warm compresses before you breastfeed can help the milk flow. Only use warmth right before breastfeeding since heat can increase inflammation.

Use cold. At other times, try cold. You can use an ice pack with crushed ice, a reusable soft ice pack, or a bag of frozen peas or corn. Wrap cold compresses in a towel to protect your skin, and apply them for fifteen to twenty minutes at a time.

Wear a supportive bra. A sports or other supportive bra can be helpful. If it feels good, you can even wear one at night. Avoid underwire bras or those that are too tight, since consistent compression on the breast can cause mastitis.

Watch for possible infection. If your temperature rises to above 100.6°F (38.4°C), and/or you are having any symptoms that feel like the flu, call your health-care provider. You may have an infection.

Use an anti-inflammatory. Ibuprofen or other anti-inflammatories can help with discomfort, and most are compatible with breastfeeding. Ask your health-care provider to recommend one.

If you follow the above suggestions, your symptoms should clear in a day or two. If they do not, don't try to tough it out. Contact skilled breastfeeding help. There could be something else going on. And remember, this too shall pass.

Nipple Pain and Trauma

Nipple pain can be very discouraging and can even make you depressed! The good news is that it *should not hurt* to breastfeed. More than a twinge at the beginning during the first week or two means that an adjustment is needed. And this isn't an invitation to beat yourself up for not being the perfect breastfeeder, just a reminder to get the help you need to make breastfeeding comfortable for you.

NIPPLE TRAUMA IS NOT NORMAL

One pervasive idea that we'd love to change is that nipple trauma is normal during breastfeeding, a common cultural belief that has undermined breastfeeding for countless mothers. Although many mothers experience some discomfort during breastfeeding at first, the only type of nipple pain that we consider normal today is very mild tenderness at the beginning of a feeding during the first week or two after birth. Nipple discomfort that is truly in this normal range subsides after a minute or two of breastfeeding, when the mother's milk is released or lets down.

Many mothers have pain well outside these normal parameters but mistakenly believe that they have to endure it until it goes away on its own. They may delay seeking help or even give up on breastfeeding entirely. Pain during breastfeeding is a common reason women wean before they had planned. Nipple pain when it is *not* normal includes:

- intense, toe-curling pain;

- pain throughout the feeding or between feedings;

- broken skin, blisters, or color changes;

- a burning sensation during, after, or in-between feedings;

- persistent soreness that does not improve after a day or two of trying to correct the problem.

Any woman experiencing any of these should seek skilled breastfeeding help immediately. Below we've listed some of the more common causes of nipple pain and what you can do about them.

SHALLOW LATCH

Shallow latch is one of the most common causes of nipple pain. Some of the telltale signs are:

- a nipple that emerges from your baby's mouth oddly shaped, with its surface at an angle, like a new tube of lipstick;

- a vertical or horizontal crease on your nipple, or a scab that develops on the face of the nipple.

Shallow latch can be caused or aggravated by engorgement or the use of bottles and pacifiers. Unusual anatomy in mother or baby, such as tongue-tie and inverted nipples, or "fit" issues will be covered later in this chapter. For any problem with latch on, review chapter 3 for suggestions on how to improve your latch.

OTHER CAUSES OF NIPPLE PAIN

Nipple pain can also be due to other problems.

Not breaking baby's suction. You can cause nipple trauma by taking your baby off your breast without first releasing the suction in his mouth. We always wince when we see moms do this. Moms of older babies sometimes find that their nipples are sore because babies turn their heads to see what is going on while still attached to Mom! To remove the baby safely, slide your little finger into the corner of your baby's mouth between his gums until he releases your breast. Then remove your breast from his mouth.

Improper use of a breast pump. A wide variety of breast pumps are on the market. Some are excellent—others are not. Some of the discount pumps can be too strong and can damage your nipples. Also, some mothers mistakenly believe that if they crank their pump to the maximum setting, it will give them even more milk. This doesn't help. A too-tight fit can cause pain, too. Never continue to use a pump if it hurts.

Cleaning products and personal-care practices. Sometimes moms get sore nipples because of overzealous cleaning. You don't need to clean your breasts before you breastfeed. Your body already does this for you. If you use a topical ointment, choose one that does not need to be wiped off before your baby breastfeeds (such as Lansinoh ultra-purified lanolin, as described in an upcoming section). Also avoid breast pads or bras with plastic liners, as these can trap moisture next to the nipple and cause skin breakdown.

Raynaud's Phenomenon. Raynaud's phenomenon involves an involuntary constriction of the arteries so that body parts (usually hands or feet) blanch or turn white, blue, and/or red. This can also happen in the nipples, and it can cause searing nipple pain. If your nipple blanches after you nurse, ask a lactation consultant or your health-care provider to evaluate it. If necessary, the prescription drug nifedipine can sometimes be helpful with Raynaud's and is compatible with breastfeeding.

Infections of the breast and skin problems. Infections can also cause severe pain. These can include mastitis and thrush (a yeast infection) and bacterial infection of the skin, as well as skin problems such as contact dermatitis, eczema, and psoriasis. These are described in more detail in the next section.

Nipple bleb. A white spot on the nipple that sometimes causes pain during breastfeeding. (See our Web site for more information.)

WHAT YOU CAN DO

There are a variety of things that you can do to eliminate nipple pain. You don't have to keep suffering in order to breastfeed your baby. You will need to continue to drain your breasts, either by breastfeeding or by pumping. Don't wean suddenly, as you will likely end up with a worse problem (see chapter 7).

Fix the latch. Make sure that your baby is latching well. Toughing it out does no one any good. And if things don't seem to be any better within a day or so, contact skilled breastfeeding help and arrange to see someone.

Offer your least sore breast first. If you have nipple trauma, try different breastfeeding positions to find one that doesn't hurt or put pressure on any tender spots until help arrives. You might also try offering your less sore breast first, and then switch to the other side after your milk lets down.

Express your milk. If your nipples are severely damaged or infected, you may prefer to rent a pump to drain your breasts until things heal up a bit. Don't use a cheap pump, or things might get worse. Some mothers find that pumping hurts less than breastfeeding. Just remember that you will need to drain your breasts at least eight times a day.

Use ultra-purified lanolin (such as Lansinoh brand) if you have trauma. It is no longer recommended to keep broken skin on your nipple dry. Lanolin provides moist wound healing, allowing your nipple to heal without forming a scab. Creating a healthy moisture balance reduces pain and speeds healing. If the friction of your clothing bothers you, use Lansinoh with breast shells (hard plastic shells worn in your bra) to prevent your nipples from touching your clothing. If you use breast shells, be sure your bra cup is large enough to accommodate them without putting pressure on your breasts.

Hydrogel dressings. A new treatment for nipple pain and trauma is hydrogel dressings (one example is the Ameda ComfortGels), a soothing gel pad worn in the bra that also provides moist wound healing to reduce pain and speed healing. In a recent study (Dodd and Chalmers 2003), hydrogel dressings decreased women's pain more than lanolin without increasing the risk of infection. Ask your lactation consultant or hospital about them.

Treat infections or skin problems. If you have a bacterial or fungal infection (see below), see your practitioner about treatment. You can continue to breastfeed while you are being treated for an infection, but in some cases (as with thrush), your baby may need to be treated, too.

Mastitis

Mastitis refers to any inflammation of the breast, with or without a fever. A mild form of mastitis—a tender spot or lump in your breast with no fever—is sometimes referred to as a *plugged duct*. If you have a temperature of more than 101°F (38.4°C), are achey, or have other symptoms that feel like the flu, you most likely have a more severe case that has progressed into an infection. Other signs of infection include a cracked nipple with pus, pus or blood in your milk, red streaks on your breast, and symptoms that appear suddenly and are severe.

WHAT YOU CAN DO

For mastitis with and without infection, the treatment is generally the same. However, if you think you have an infection, call your health-care provider and ask about a prescription of antibiotics, and then follow the suggestions we describe below.

Breastfeed frequently on the affected breast. Drain the affected breast frequently with a baby and/or a pump. Allowing milk to accumulate in your breast will make matters worse. You may hesitate to breastfeed because it is uncomfortable. If so, try different positions until you find the one that is most comfortable. You might also talk with your health-care provider about using an over-the-counter medication, such as ibuprofen, to lessen your symptoms and to help with pain. If your baby refuses to nurse on your affected side, you may need to pump on that side until the infection heals.

Apply heat to the area and gently massage it. Massage the area with your palm and fingers in a circular motion. You can also use your fingertips to knead your breast. Move from your armpit to your nipple. You can also soak your breast in warm water in a bath, or leaning over a basin. Do this at least three times a day.

Breastfeed your baby immediately after you treat with heat. This will help loosen the plug.

Wear loose clothing. Avoid tight or restrictive clothing while healing mastitis. Also consider whether your bra is too tight. A tight bra can actually cause mastitis.

Rest. Mastitis may be your body's way of telling you that you are doing too much. Be sure to rest as much as you can to allow your body's natural defenses to fight any possible infection. Mothers who have recurrent cases of mastitis are often the ones who are running themselves ragged.

Consider possible causes. Your key to avoiding another case of mastitis may be to determine why you got it in the first place. Two common causes are broken skin on the nipple and a bra that's too tight. Another is anything that allows the breast to become overly full, such as irregular feeding patterns, a sudden change (such as when your baby begins sleeping through the night), the use of supplements, bottles, or a pacifier, or lengthening the times between feedings. Too-full breasts can also happen at times when you're really busy and go longer between feedings (holidays and family get-togethers can be key times). If any of these situations apply to you, do what you can to change them to help avoid a recurrence of your symptoms. And remember, sudden weaning can make matters worse.

Thrush/Yeast Infections

Another type of possible infection is caused by yeast or *Candida albicans*. Yeast infections can be painful for both mothers and babies. Your baby can have a yeast infection, which will appear as white patches inside his mouth (*thrush*) or as diaper rash.

Your baby may have a yeast infection if he has diaper rash, discomfort in his mouth at feedings, white patches in his mouth, or a white tongue (he does not have to have all of these symptoms). You may have a yeast infection if you have nipple pain that is burning or shooting (rather than stabbing or pinching, as from other causes). You may have redness, scaling, or flaking, or the skin of the areola may be smooth and shiny. Or your breasts may not look different at all. The pain may begin after a period of pain-free breastfeeding and may be quite severe. Your nipples may or may not be itchy. It may be worse after feeding or at night. *Candida albicans can cause nipple pain even if no thrush is seen in baby's mouth.*

If you have a yeast infection on your nipples, it's important for you to treat both yourself and your baby. Yeast is contagious. Unless you both are treated, you are likely to reinfect each other. You may also need to treat any other family members (including your partner) if they have symptoms of yeast.

TREATMENT OPTIONS

The following are treatment options for your baby. Work with your health-care provider to find the best medication for you to use. Treatments for your baby include nystatin suspension (which has become much less effective in recent years due to its common usage, leading to the spread of nystatin-resistant strains of thrush), gentian violet, clotrimazole, and fluconazole.

Treatment options for you include nystatin cream or ointment; gentian violet; over-the-counter antifungal creams such as clotrimazole (sold as Mycelex, Lotrimin, Lotrimin AF cream or lotion [1%]), miconazole (sold as Mycatin, Monistat-Derm cream or lotion [2%]), and ketoconazole (sold as Nizoral); nystatin with triamcinolone (a corticosteroid), and Dr. Jack Newman's All Purpose Nipple Ointment. For more specific information, see our Web site.

If you have deep breast pain, it may or may not be due to yeast. More commonly, deep breast pain is due to a bacterial infection of the nipple or Raynaud's phenomenon (see the earlier section "Other Causes of Nipple Pain"). Contact your health-care provider or lactation specialist for further help.

Low Milk Supply

Low milk supply is the most common reason mothers give for premature weaning. Sometimes, a mother's milk supply is not low at all. She only thinks that it is. If you are not sure, review chapters 4 and 5. These will give you some specific guidelines on what is normal and how to tell whether your baby is getting enough milk. If after reviewing these chapters, you decide that you need to increase your milk supply—or if your baby has been losing or not gaining weight— here are some techniques to help you make more milk.

Breastfeed more. Try to feed at least eight to twelve times per day, and drain the breasts more fully each time. As we described in chapter 6, the more times per day that milk is effectively removed, the faster your milk supply will increase. Focus on the *number of feedings per day,* not the time between feedings (commonly, every two or three hours). Encourage the baby to breastfeed whenever he shows feeding cues, such as rooting, hand to mouth, or fussing, even if it has only been a short time since he last ate. To drain more milk each time, use each breast more than once and express milk after feedings (see next point).

Work to improve baby's latch. Review chapter 3 to help improve the baby's latch. A more effective latch will help your baby remove more milk from your breast, thereby signaling your body to make more.

Stimulate a sleepy baby. If your baby stops nursing actively or falls asleep within ten minutes at breast, stimulate baby to breastfeed actively for longer using breast compression and by switching breasts (see the section "Sleepy Baby" later in this chapter).

Pump with a rental pump. Double pump (pump both breasts at the same time) for ten to fifteen minutes either right after feedings or after about half an hour. The more times per day the breasts are effectively drained, the more milk production is increased. If possible, pump long enough so that two minutes pass after you see the last drop of milk, or pump twenty to thirty minutes, whichever comes first. This has been found to increase milk supply faster.

Decrease supplementation. If your baby is younger than one month, consider supplementing with a feeding method other than bottles, such as a nursing supplementer, cup, syringe, or spoon (see chapter 11). Gradually decrease the supplementation as your milk supply increases.

Try herbs or other medications to increase milk. The herb fenugreek is another way to increase your supply. Fenugreek has a long history of use as a *galactagogue,* or substance that increases milk production, and the U.S. Food and Drug Administration has given it a rating of GRAS (generally recognized as safe). However, it can interact with a few prescription and over-the-counter medications and should be discussed with your health-care provider before you take it (Hale 2004; Humphrey 2003). Take three capsules (of at least 500 mg each) three times per day (nine total per day). This is a higher dose than is on the label because label dosages are not for increasing milk. You can buy fenugreek at health food stores.

Two prescription medications that increase milk production are metoclopramide (Reglan) and domperidone (Motilium). Both are drugs normally prescribed for stomach problems. Studies indicate that metoclopramide and domperidone can increase milk supply. Domperidone is currently under an FDA ban in the U.S., and is therefore not available at this writing. It is currently available in other countries, however, and is highly effective (see our Web site for updated information). Since depression can be a side effect of metoclopramide, you may want to avoid it if you have a history of depression (Hale 2004). Talk to your doctor about it.

Overabundant Milk Supply

Mothers can also have too much milk. While this is a better problem to have than too little milk, it still can cause difficulties. Too much milk can be mighty unpleasant for your baby. To understand how he feels, think what it would be like for you if someone were to pour a quart of liquid into your mouth, giving you no way to control the flow. Overabundance can be why babies will sometimes push away from the breast, pull back or clamp down on the nipple, or refuse to breastfeed altogether. Some signs that indicate that you may have too much milk include the following:

- Your baby is gaining much more than 2 pounds (907 g) per month.

- He has trouble keeping up with the flow of your milk, and he gulps, chokes, or sputters when he nurses.

- He seems unusually gassy or has frothy or explosive stools.

This last point, in and of itself, does not indicate an overabundant milk supply, but when seen in combination with an unusually large weight gain, it may be another clue.

WHAT YOU CAN DO

Fortunately, there are some simple things that you can do to help your baby cope with your abundance of milk. The most straightforward technique is to limit each feeding session to only one breast. That way, your baby gets more of the fattier hindmilk available in the latter part of the feeding session. Your baby will feel more satisfied because he has gotten more calories. If needed, you can pump to comfort on the other side, but you don't want to completely drain your breast since this will signal your body to keep making lots of milk. Try this for four to seven days to see if your baby's symptoms improve.

Use one breast for more than one feeding. If your baby is still having difficulty coping, or you have a forceful letdown, there are some other techniques that you can try. Use the same breast for two or three feedings in a row, pumping the other breast to comfort as needed. If you have a very large oversupply, this can help your body adjust more rapidly.

Try different positions. One position to try is having your baby sit on your thigh (one leg hanging over each side), facing your breast. Support his back and head. Or try lying flat on your back and having your baby lie on top of you to breastfeed. That way, gravity slows the flow of milk. You might also find that the side-lying position works well for you because your baby can let milk dribble out of his mouth, rather than feeling like he needs to swallow to keep from choking.

Other options. You can also try starting the flow of your milk by hand expressing or using a pump. When the flow of milk has slowed somewhat, then put the baby to breast. Other mothers have found that a nipple shield (a flexible silicone nipple worn over your breast during feedings, used for a few days or weeks) can help babies cope with the flow of their mothers' milk. Frequent nursings can also help since less milk will have accumulated in the breast, making it easier for your baby to cope.

As a final caution, be sure that you never hold your baby's head to your breast to make sure that he breastfeeds. If your baby feels like he's choking, your holding his head there can make him not want to go anywhere near your breast, even when really hungry. Again, think how you would feel if someone was forcing a quart of liquid down your throat. If you allow your baby to have some control over how much he takes in during each suck/swallow sequence, your baby's time at your breast will be much more pleasant for both of you.

BABY-RELATED CHALLENGES

The following are some challenges that relate more to your baby than to you.

Sleepy Baby

Most newborns need to feed eight to twelve times per twenty-four hours to gain and grow well. But some babies don't know this. You may need to awaken your baby to feed more often or for a longer time if he:

- has lost more than 10 percent of his birth weight in the first three to four days;

- is not gaining at least 4 to 5 ounces (113 to 142 g) per week after day four;

- is falling asleep before at least ten to fifteen minutes of good, active sucking on the first breast during the first week of life;

- has fewer than three to four good-sized stools per twenty-four hours (this is not a problem if weight gain is good);

- is jaundiced.

TO INCREASE THE NUMBER OF FEEDINGS

To increase the number of times your baby feeds per day, you may need to wake him for some feedings. To do this, first make sure your baby is not too warm. As your baby gets warmer, sleepiness increases and active sucking decreases. Dress your baby in the same weight clothing that you would wear and even lighter when breastfeeding, as your body heat will warm him, too. Before trying to wake him up, wait until he is in a light sleep cycle. He's in a light sleep cycle if his eyes are moving under his eyelids, or if his mouth or any other body part is moving. Babies pass in and out of deep sleep often. Just wait.

The doll's-eye technique. When your baby is ready to wake, try the "doll's-eye" technique below:

- Lay your baby in your lap facing up, with his head at your knees and his feet at your torso.

- Put your thumbs under your baby's armpits and your fingers behind his head.

- Do "baby sit-ups" by laying baby down flat in your lap and sitting him up.

- Don't do this too slowly, as it can make your baby sleepy rather than rousing him.

- Some babies will rouse (root, open their eyes, act agitated) after only a few sit-ups, while others will take several minutes.

TO INCREASE THE LENGTH OF FEEDINGS

Increasing the number of feedings will not help if the baby still falls asleep at the breast before getting enough milk. Here are some techniques to help increase the amount of time babies spend breastfeeding actively.

Work to improve baby's latch. This will ensure that your baby gets a faster milk flow to better keep him interested (see chapter 3).

Breast compression. This technique was popularized by pediatrician Jack Newman, MD. It increases the flow of milk to the baby, keeping him interested and feeding actively for longer. Leave your baby on the first breast to "finish" before switching breasts. As Dr. Newman writes: "How do you know the baby is finished? When he no longer drinks at the breast (open mouth wide–pause–then close mouth type of suck)" (Newman and Pitman 2000, pp. 82–3). To do breast compression:

1. Hold the baby with one arm and hold your breast with the opposite hand.

2. Position your thumb on one side of the breast and your other fingers on the other, well away from the nipple and areola (the dark area around your nipple).

3. Watch for the wide jaw movements that tell you your baby is getting milk. The baby gets more milk when he is drinking with an open mouth wide–pause–close mouth type of suck. (Open mouth wide–pause–close mouth is one suck; the pause is not a pause between sucks.)

4. When the baby is nibbling or no longer drinking with the open mouth wide–pause–close mouth type of suck, compress the breast. Not so hard that it hurts, and try not to change the shape of the breast near the baby's mouth. With the compression, the baby should start drinking again with the open mouth wide–pause–close mouth type of suck.

5. Keep the pressure up (don't stop compressing) until the baby is no longer drinking milk actively even with the compression, then release the pressure. Often the baby will stop sucking when the pressure is released but will start again shortly as milk starts to flow. If the baby does not stop sucking with the release of pressure, wait a short time before compressing again.

6. The reason to release the pressure is to allow your hand to rest and to allow milk to start flowing to the baby again. The

baby, if he stops sucking when you release the pressure, will start again when he starts to taste milk.

7. When the baby starts sucking again, he may drink (open mouth wide–pause–close mouth). If not, compress again as above.

8. Continue on the first side until the baby does not drink even with the compression. You should allow the baby to stay on this side for a short time longer, as you may occasionally get another milk release and the baby will start drinking again on his own. If the baby no longer drinks, however, allow him to come off or take him off the breast. Breast compression is usually not needed for more than a few days if it is done consistently at every feeding. The baby will learn to stay active without help, although some pauses are always normal.

Switch breasts. When breast compression no longer works to keep your baby active, break the suction and take your baby off the breast. Use the doll's-eye technique (or lay him on his back on a firm surface) until he is rooting and agitated. Then put him to the other breast. Repeat as many times as needed until baby is done.

There are a few other things that you can try to wake your baby to breastfeed. You can try different breastfeeding positions, rub your baby's feet, undress him, or change his diaper. Once your baby starts taking more milk, he will perk up and these techniques won't be necessary.

Exaggerated Newborn Jaundice

Babies are born with extra red blood cells. These extra cells break down in the early weeks of life, producing a substance called *bilirubin*. When there is too much bilirubin in your baby's blood, he becomes jaundiced and his skin takes on a yellow hue. Jaundice is a common condition, occurring in more than half of all newborns (Mohrbacher and Stock 2003). Although this puts newborn jaundice in the "normal" category, jaundice is important for your baby's doctor to monitor since it can lead to more serious conditions if it becomes severe.

Finding out that your baby has exaggerated jaundice can be frightening. And sometimes, steps taken to correct it can interfere with breastfeeding. The standard advice used to be that mothers should stop breastfeeding so their babies could be treated. However, research has revealed that breastfeeding actually helps resolve jaundice. So in most cases, you should continue breastfeeding without interruption.

DIFFERENT TYPES OF JAUNDICE

There are different types of jaundice, and some require no treatment. One way that doctors tell the difference between the types of jaundice is by the timing of the first symptoms. If the jaundice appears on the first day, it generally indicates a physical cause unrelated to feeding, such as Rh and ABO blood compatibilities, liver enzyme deficiency diseases, or conditions such as gastrointestinal obstructions. With rare exceptions, breastfeeding should proceed normally.

Jaundice that appears on days two to five is more common, occurring in about half of all newborns. Some babies, such as those of Asian, Native American/American Indian, or South American ethnicity normally have higher levels of bilirubin. Unless baby's bilirubin reaches unsafe levels, normal newborn jaundice tends to resolve on its own within a few days or weeks, especially if the baby is feeding eight to twelve times in twenty-four hours and is passing stools. Indeed, effective breastfeeding (at least nine to eleven times per day from birth in one study) prevents exaggerated bilirubin levels (levels higher than 15 mg/dl; Yamauchi and Yamanouchi 1990).

Colostrum, the early milk, also acts as a natural laxative and helps the baby eliminate bilirubin through his stools. If babies don't receive enough colostrum in the first few days, the meconium, the black tarry stool, may not be passed, and the bilirubin in the meconium will be reabsorbed into their bloodstream (causing bilirubin levels to rise). Babies at risk for exaggerated jaundice are those who are not feeding well. Those at higher risk are babies born "near-term" (thirty-five to thirty-eight weeks gestation), who are often sent home from the hospital not feeding well. Exaggerated newborn jaundice is one common reason for these babies to be readmitted to the hospital.

Jaundice can even appear after the baby's first week. There is a condition called "late-onset" or "breast-milk" jaundice that researchers are discovering may be more common than previously believed. It may affect up to one-third of babies. Indeed, researchers are beginning to speculate that this might be the normal pattern, rather than the abnormally low level of bilirubin found in formula-fed babies. As long as bilirubin levels are not in the pathological range (generally above 20 mg/dl), this condition will generally resolve on its own without treatment.

One difficulty of jaundice is that it tends to make babies sleepy. Moms sometimes don't realize that anything is amiss, only that their babies seem to sleep a lot. Unfortunately, these babies are often the ones who are not feeding well simply because they are not breastfeeding enough times during the day. Moreover, these babies may fall asleep at the breast before they've had enough milk. The result is poor weight gain and bilirubin levels that are too high. See suggestions in the previous section for coaxing a sleepy baby to eat.

TREATMENTS FOR JAUNDICE

Fortunately for mothers and babies, strategies recommended for jaundice have changed in recent years to encourage breastfeeding. In most cases, as long as breastfeeding is going well, a mother should continue breastfeeding with health-care providers checking baby's bilirubin level from time to time. Effective breastfeeding should guarantee the passage of many stools per day, which is the primary way baby clears the bilirubin from his system. You should also avoid giving your baby water supplements since these slow the clearance of bilirubin by cutting down on the number of times that babies breastfeed and stool during the day.

In previous times, the standard protocol for treatment of jaundice was to use formula. Fortunately, this is no longer true. However, there are some times when formula is called for. If your milk supply is low, you may need to use formula for a few feedings to increase the number of stools that your baby has. However, while doing this, you can start pumping your breasts to increase your milk supply. Any expressed milk that you have can be given to your baby.

Your doctor may want your baby to receive phototherapy. Phototherapy may involve either placing the baby under lights or using a special wrap that helps break down bilirubin through the skin. If lights are used, your baby will be placed under them wearing only a diaper and some protective patches on his eyes. You may be able to rent phototherapy equipment to provide treatment at home. If your baby is rehospitalized, you may be able to stay in the nursery with your baby or have the bililights set up in your hospital room. When your baby seems hungry, you can remove him from the lights, breastfeed him, and then return him to the lights, as the lights do not need to be used continuously to be effective. With proper management, the jaundice should safely clear in a few days or weeks without compromising breastfeeding. See our Web site for the American Academy of Pediatrics treatment guidelines that you can share with your baby's doctor.

Breast Refusal or Nursing Strike

A baby who refuses to breastfeed can be devastating for any mom. Your baby may refuse the breast as a newborn, or he may suddenly refuse to breastfeed after several weeks or months of breastfeeding well. This is called a nursing strike.

It's very easy to think that your baby doesn't like *you* or your milk, and your baby's behavior can feel like a personal rejection. If you are feeling that way, we can totally sympathize. However, we also want to reassure you that your baby is *not* making a judgment about you. It's true that your baby may not like breastfeeding—at the moment. But your baby prefers you to all other people. He recognizes the sound of your voice, the smell of your body, the unique taste of your milk. Just smelling or hearing you reassures him. So what we need to focus on right now is how to make breastfeeding a more pleasurable experience for you both. Unfortunately, when you feel rejected, it takes you out of problem-solving mode. So we ask that, for the moment, you try to see this from the baby's perspective. That will often suggest a solution.

TRY TO LOCATE A CAUSE

When dealing with a nursing strike, or refusal to breastfeed, locating the possible cause can be helpful. It would probably be a good time for you to call a lactation consultant or a mother-to-mother breastfeeding counselor in your area to see if the two of you can figure this out. If no one is available, we'll give you some suggestions on where to start.

Did your baby have an injury at birth or might he be in pain? Sometimes babies refuse the breast because they are uncomfortable when held in a certain position. If your baby's mouth was roughly suctioned at birth, he may have a sore throat or be afraid to allow anything into his mouth. If you suspect that this might be the case, try various positions to see if one is more comfortable for you and your baby. Try the hardwiring ideas in chapter 1 to help your baby feel more at ease when held close.

Do you have a forceful letdown? In a previous section, we discussed what happens when your baby is trying to cope with too much milk all at once. See "Overabundant Milk Supply" earlier in this chapter for some suggestions about how to cope with this.

Have you or someone else been trying to force your baby to breastfeed? This can happen when well-meaning moms or helpers decide to force the baby to the breast. Your baby may get to the point where he wants nothing to do with it.

Does your baby have a good latch? Babies who have a poor latch-on to the breast are not able to keep up a good milk flow. This can be frustrating for them. Review chapter 3 for suggestions.

Is your baby getting enough milk when he feeds? Sometimes breastfeeding, especially early on, is frustrating for babies when they are really hungry and there is little or no food. If your supply is low and/or your baby is very hungry, your baby may find that nursing isn't much fun.

Is your baby ill or has he been biting? A baby may refuse to breastfeed when he has an ear infection (which makes breastfeeding painful) or a cold. You may want to see your baby's health-care provider to rule out a physical problem. If your baby has bitten you and you startled him by jumping or yelling (an understandable reaction!), that can sometimes cause a baby to temporarily refuse the breast.

Has something changed in your life? Babies sometimes react to a prolonged separation or unusual stress in the family by refusing the breast.

WHAT YOU CAN DO

Fortunately, there are some steps you can take to help coax your baby back onto the breast.

- *Have lots of contact with your baby.* Review chapter 2 and have lots of skin-to-skin contact with your baby. Carry your baby. Sleep with him. Offer the breast when he's in a quiet, alert state but not necessarily hungry. Make the breast a pleasant place to be.

- *Try breastfeeding when your baby is asleep or half asleep.* Many babies will breastfeed without thinking if they are not fully awake.

- *Watch for early hunger cues.* Mothers can have difficulties when they wait until their babies are frantically hungry before feeding them. As we described earlier, your baby will be a lot more cooperative if he is not famished.

- *Take advantage of your baby's hardwiring.* See chapters 1 and 2 for ways to calm and relax your baby. Your baby is born wanting to breastfeed. Use his natural responses to help make it happen.

- *Feed the baby and protect your supply.* The refusal to nurse can take a few days to resolve. In the meantime, you need to protect your supply and feed your baby. See chapter 11 for suggestions on preserving your milk supply with a pump. You may also need to feed your baby either your pumped milk or some supplementary formula if your milk supply is low. Just keep in mind that the goal is to return your baby happily to the breast.

- *Get help.* Don't hesitate to get skilled breastfeeding help if you're not making progress on your own.

You and your baby can overcome breast refusal or a nursing strike. Get support and have patience. It's well worth the extra effort.

CHAPTER 11

Special Situations: Physical or Health Issues

Sometimes breastfeeding can be challenging because of illness or an ongoing physical issue. In this chapter, we describe some strategies you can use if you encounter difficulties in your own or your baby's health that are influencing breastfeeding.

SPECIAL SITUATIONS: MOTHER

Many mothers worry that breastfeeding may be compromised if they have an acute or chronic illness, if they are depressed or have other emotional issues, or if there is something unusual about their anatomy. That's what this section is about. We want you to know up front that there are few reasons to wean, even temporarily. In most cases, breast-feeding will still be your and your baby's best bet.

Acute or Chronic Illness

Illness can take many forms. It can be temporary, or it can be a long-standing health concern. In this section, we address how acute and chronic illness and other physical conditions can influence breastfeeding. We'll also offer suggestions on what you can do.

FLU OR COLD

When you have a cold or the flu, you may be concerned about infecting your baby. It's important to know that breastfeeding is the only protection your baby has from your illness. Once you have symptoms, your baby has already been exposed, because you are most contagious just before your symptoms appear. One of the first things your body does is to produce specific antibodies to fight that illness, some of which go right into your milk. If your baby continues breastfeeding, the antibodies in your milk will either prevent her from catching the illness, or if she does get sick, she'll get a milder case. If you stop breastfeeding now, your baby will be deprived of the only available protection.

Breastfeeding during your illness also may be helpful for you. While you are sick, you can simply tuck your baby into bed with you and not have to worry about getting up to prepare bottles, or worse, going to the store to buy formula. Breastfeeding gives you a way of caring for your baby even when you can do little else.

When you're sick, be sure to drink enough fluids to prevent dehydration, which in severe cases can temporarily affect your milk production. If you are too sick to breastfeed for a few days, see the section in this chapter for suggestions on what to do if you must temporarily stop breastfeeding.

Chronic Health Problems

Chronic health problems are relatively common. If you have a chronic illness, you may have concerns about breastfeeding. Below we describe several common conditions and offer specific suggestions to you. But we also have some general advice.

GENERAL SUGGESTIONS FOR MOTHERS WITH CHRONIC ILLNESS

The following guidelines may seem like common sense, but when you're adjusting to caring for an infant while also dealing with a chronic illness, it's good to be reminded to take care of yourself.

Make sure you get enough rest. Fatigue is common for new mothers and even more so for mothers with chronic illnesses. It is essential that you rest regularly. That's where Laws 2, 4, and 5 (use skin-to-skin, breastfeed frequently, and follow your own feeding rhythm) will be particularly useful. Nap with your baby. Hold your baby skin to skin during the day. Learn to nurse lying down so that you can rest during the day. Keep your baby close at night so that you don't need to fully wake up to attend to your baby's needs. And limit the number of guests that you have (especially those you have to entertain).

Accept all offers of help. So often new mothers think that they need to handle everything alone. This is not the time to demonstrate your independence. Being overly fatigued can cause your symptoms to flare. So for the first few weeks or more, accept help.

Get advice about your medications. You might be currently taking one or more prescription medications. Most medications are compatible with breastfeeding, but a few are not. Check with your local La Leche League leader, Australian Breastfeeding Association counselor, or lactation consultant, who generally will have access to reference materials that other health-care providers do not. Another option is to purchase your own copy of *Medications and Mothers' Milk* (see our Resources section or Web site for order information).

Realize that you may be vulnerable to depression. Several types of chronic illness are associated with higher risks of depression (for instance, lupus, rheumatoid arthritis, MS). Be aware that you are probably more vulnerable than most mothers. If you seek support and follow the steps listed above, you have a good chance of preventing an occurrence of depression.

INFLAMMATORY ARTHRITIS, MULTIPLE SCLEROSIS, AND MYASTHENIA GRAVIS

Several kinds of chronic illness are more common for women of childbearing age. These include the various types of inflammatory arthritis (such a lupus, rheumatoid arthritis, or systemic sclerosis) and other illnesses such as multiple sclerosis (MS) and myasthenia gravis (MG). All of these illnesses can cause muscle weakness, pain, and swelling. Indeed, having a baby may actually trigger a flare-up of symptoms in the first few months postpartum. But it is still better for you to breast-feed. Your baby cannot "catch" your illness through breastfeeding, as these illnesses are caused by a combination of genetics and environmental factors. Indeed, breastfeeding may protect your baby from ever contracting one of them. Below are some suggestions for coping.

Support your upper-body joints. You will need to find a position that allows you to hold your baby comfortably while not stressing your upper-body joints. Keep a variety of pillows and other supports available so that you don't stress your hands, wrists, elbows, shoulders, or neck.

Watch how you carry your baby. Carrying your baby can also stress your joints and muscles. Front-packs can stress your neck and shoulders. A baby sling is helpful because it takes the stress off your shoulders, wrists, and hands. These are available from many local hospitals or you can find them online (see our Web site for more information). Cuddling your baby while you are sitting or lying down allows you to connect with her in a way that doesn't stress your joints and muscles. You might want to ask your physical therapist about some exercises and stretches to counter some of the strain of carrying your baby.

You *can* care for a baby, even with a chronic illness. Pace yourself, get help and support, and take whatever medications you feel are necessary. See our Web site for more information.

DIABETES

Diabetes is a metabolic disorder caused by your body's inability to make enough insulin or to use the insulin that is available (insulin resistance). If you are diabetic, breastfeeding offers you several important advantages. Generally speaking, diabetes is easier to manage during breastfeeding, as you may require less insulin. And if you had gestational diabetes, breastfeeding can prevent the development of diabetes when you're not pregnant. Even with these advantages, there are some special considerations for the diabetic mother.

Increased risk of hypoglycemia in your baby. About half of all babies born to diabetic mothers have hypoglycemia, or low blood sugar. This may require some intervention while you are in the hospital.

You may experience a delay in your milk increasing. Some diabetic mothers experience a one-to-four-day delay in when their milk "comes in." Breastfeeding early and often will help. Even with a delay, you can bring in a full supply.

You may need extra calories. While you breastfeed, you may need extra calories to help you maintain an adequate supply. When breast-feeding is established, you may need to adjust how much you eat depending on whether the baby is breastfeeding a little or a lot. You may also need to adjust your dosage of insulin based on how much your baby is breastfeeding. This should be obvious as you monitor your blood-sugar levels.

Be alert to possible infections. As a woman with diabetes, you are more prone to all types of infections. (See our sections "Mastitis" and "Thrush/Yeast Infections" in chapter 10).

Wean gradually. As described in chapter 7, gradual weaning is best for mother and baby. For mothers with diabetes, it is also important because of the impact on your blood sugar levels. Gradual weaning will make it easier to keep your diabetes under control.

THYROID DISEASE

The thyroid is a gland that releases a hormone that regulates metabolism. Thyroid levels can be too low or too high. If you have thyroid disease, you should be under a doctor's care. If you suspect that you have it, discuss it with your health-care provider. Fortunately, in most cases you can continue to breastfeed while being treated.

Symptoms of hypothyroidism, or a low level of thyroid hormone, include extreme fatigue, inability to tolerate cold, weight gain, low basal body temperature, dry skin, thinning hair, and depression. You can develop hypothyroidism for the first time in the postpartum period. While postpartum hypothyroidism is relatively uncommon, if you have diabetes you are three times more likely to develop it (Weetman 1997).

Low thyroid can also decrease your milk supply, but thyroid supplements are compatible with breastfeeding. And if you take supplements to bring your thyroid to normal levels, you may find that it also increases your milk supply.

Hyperthyroidism refers to an overactive thyroid, which results in too-high levels of thyroid hormone in your system. This is a serious medical condition that requires prompt treatment. Most common medications used to treat hyperthyroidism are compatible with breastfeeding. However, radioactive iodine used for diagnosis or treatment is one of the few medications that breastfeeding mothers should not use. If you take this, you must wean for at least forty-eight hours, or permanently if you require longer or ongoing treatment. Radioactive materials accumulate in your milk and are passed on to the baby.

Unusual Breast or Nipple Anatomy

Every woman is unique. And not surprisingly, there is an amazing diversity of breast sizes and shapes. The overwhelming majority of breasts work just fine. But as with every other organ in the body, sometimes breasts don't function as they should. Some women encounter challenges when they have unusual nipple anatomy or there is not enough milk-producing glandular tissue to allow them to make a full milk supply. These situations are described below.

FLAT OR INVERTED NIPPLES

A flat nipple is one that does not protrude or become erect when stimulated or cold. By following Law 3 and using good latch-on technique (see our Web site for animation that shows this in motion), flat nipples should not cause breastfeeding problems, especially if at first your baby receives only the breast and is given the chance to learn to breastfeed well for several weeks before receiving bottles or pacifiers.

An inverted nipple is one that when stimulated looks like it is inside out. In most cases of inverted nipples, babies can breastfeed just fine. Again, Law 3 and good technique are important here. But if a mother has severely inverted nipples, depending on the type and the degree of inversion, breastfeeding may be difficult or impossible. Sometimes mothers have only one flat or inverted nipple, and their babies tend to prefer the other breast.

It's important to remember that babies "breastfeed" not "nipple feed." If the baby gets a good off-center latch, taking in a good amount of the areola (the pigmented area around your nipple), flat or inverted nipples will not be a problem in most cases. A nipple shield (a flexible silicone nipple with holes in the end worn over the breast during feedings) may be helpful if your baby is having difficulties getting a good latch. If you are having trouble, contact a lactation specialist for assistance. They have specialized tools, like nipple shields, and know special techniques that can usually help.

INADEQUATE GLANDULAR TISSUE

About 1 in 1,000 women have difficulty establishing a full milk supply because they do not have enough milk-producing glandular tissue in their breasts. Women who have this condition often have unusually shaped breasts. Your breasts may look tubular (long and slim) rather than rounded, may be very different in size, and your areolas may appear unusual and "bulbous." Your breasts may be widely spaced (more than 1.5 inches/3.8 cm apart), and/or did not change size at all when you were pregnant. And you may not have felt any fullness after your milk became more plentiful in the first few days postpartum. That being said, you should know that some women who have all these features have been able to establish full milk supplies. But if your baby is not gaining well, you can try the techniques we suggest to increase your milk supply (see chapter 10). Or you may need to supplement with formula. Remember, some breastfeeding is always better than none.

FIT ISSUES

Sometimes, there is a mismatch between the size of a mother's nipples and the size of her baby's mouth, especially if the mother's nipples are very large and the baby's mouth is very small. In this case, at first it may be difficult or impossible for your baby to latch on well to your breast. This can frustrate both mom and baby. If you are experiencing this, take heart. It's a problem that is quickly outgrown, usually during the first month. Once your baby's mouth grows enough, which happens very fast with a newborn, she will be able to latch on and breastfeed. In the meantime, you can establish a full milk supply with an effective, rental breast pump and feed your baby your milk (see the last section in this chapter for details).

Breast Surgery

Breast surgery is a relatively common procedure in the U.S. and in other parts of the world. You may have had a biopsy to test for cancer or remove a cyst, or you may have had a breast augmentation or reduction. And you may be concerned about whether this surgery will keep you from full breastfeeding. The answer is, as with so many other factors, it depends. Here are some general considerations.

Location of incisions. Where your breast was cut can make a tremendous difference in whether you will be able to establish a full milk supply. Generally speaking, if your surgery involved cutting around the areola, it is more likely to affect breastfeeding, as this involves cutting milk ducts and the nerves leading to the nipple. Most critical are the major nerves located at four o'clock and eight o'clock on the areola.

Surgical technique used. The technique that the surgeon used can also make a difference. If the technique leaves the milk ducts and nerves still attached to the nipple, then your odds of fully breastfeeding are greater. If these are cut, it may be more difficult. If you are reading this before you have surgery, be sure to talk with your surgeon about your desire to breastfeed. They may be able to use a technique that minimizes damage to your nerves and ducts.

Learning as much as you can about breastfeeding, no matter what type of surgery you've had, is going to be your best strategy. Some women who, biologically speaking, shouldn't have been able to breastfeed have been able to, because milk ducts can grow back after surgery. The best way for you to know whether you can breastfeed is for you to give it a try. That being said, it's important for you to know the signs of when your baby is getting enough milk so you'll know if you will need to supplement. Review chapter 4 on how to tell if your baby is getting enough milk. Weigh her frequently, either at your health-care provider's office or by renting an accurate electronic baby scale for the first few weeks postpartum. After the initial weight loss from birth to day four, your baby should gain on average about 6 ounces (170 g) a week. Also, keep track of the number of stools, as these are good indicators of how much milk your baby is getting. If your supply is low, review the section in chapter 10 about how to increase your supply.

BREAST AUGMENTATION

Breast augmentation surgery is a relatively common procedure that increases breast size by implanting silicone- or saline-filled implants under the surface of the breast, either above or below the muscles. The incisions can be under the folds in the breasts or near the armpits. These types of incisions are the least likely to have a negative impact on breastfeeding, as they usually leave the milk ducts intact. Incisions around the areola are more likely to interfere with breastfeeding. But even in this situation, some women have established full milk supplies.

Will silicone harm my baby? Some mothers with silicone implants worry that the implants may leak and silicone will get into their milk. They wonder if formula is a safer choice. If you have this concern, you may be interested to learn that both formula and cow's milk have *ten times* more silicone than the milk of mothers with implants (Mohrbacher and Stock 2003). In addition, silicone itself is considered inert, so even if your baby did ingest some, her digestive tract is unlikely to absorb it. In fact, one form of silicone (simethicone) is given directly to babies as a commonly used colic treatment. So, as usual, you're better off breastfeeding.

BREAST REDUCTION

Breast reduction is another relatively common procedure where fat and tissue are removed from the breast. Unfortunately, this procedure almost always involves cutting at least some of the milk ducts. The more tissue you have removed, the less likely you will be able to establish a full milk supply. Your chances decrease further if your surgery involved removing the nipple and relocating it to a different place on the breast. However, there is at least one case report of a woman who did bring in a full supply with both of these factors. This is rare, but not out of the realm of possibility. With time, some severed milk ducts grow back. So the best approach is for you to try breastfeeding while keeping track of how much your baby is getting. Even if you bring in a partial milk supply, some breastfeeding is better than none. If you would like to know more about breastfeeding after reduction, we suggest that you get a copy of Diana West's 2001 book *Defining Your Own Success: Breastfeeding After Breast Reduction Surgery* (see our Resource list or Web site for ordering information or go to her Web site, www.bfar.org.).

Depression, Difficult Birth, Past Sexual Abuse

You may be surprised to learn that your emotional health can have an impact on breastfeeding. In this section, we describe three factors that relate to emotional well-being, and how these can impact your breastfeeding relationship.

DEPRESSION

Depression in the postpartum period is relatively common, affecting 10 to 20 percent of new mothers in Western cultures. The percentages of depressed mothers can be even higher in some high-risk populations. Some of the common symptoms of postpartum depression include sadness, hopelessness, an inability to experience pleasure from everyday activities, excessive emotional sensitivity, sleep and appetite disturbances (too much or too little), agitation, irritability, and an inability to concentrate. It's normal to have some of these symptoms for a day or two. But if they persist for at least two weeks, you might be suffering from depression according to the *Diagnostic and Statistical Manual of Mental Disorders-IV* (American Psychiatric Association 2000).

Depression in new mothers can be caused by a whole range of factors. These can be broken down into roughly five categories: physiological factors, such as pain and fatigue; negative birth experiences (see next section); infant characteristics, such as temperament, prematurity, and disability; psychological factors, such as self-esteem and previous episodes of depression; and social factors, such as childhood loss and abuse, lack of support, and low income (Kendall-Tackett 2005). Much more information is available on our Web site. If you are depressed, there are a couple of things that are important for you to keep in mind.

Depression can cause you to quit breastfeeding. Several recent studies have found that depressed mothers quit breastfeeding significantly earlier than nondepressed mothers. Knowing this can help you persevere.

Depression can influence how you relate to your baby. Dozens of studies have documented that depression can have a negative impact on how you respond to your baby. Depressed mothers are often not as tuned-in to their babies' cues, they are not as positive when interacting with their babies, and they make eye contact less often. One recent study found that breastfeeding helped protect babies from the negative effects of their mothers' depression (Jones et al. 2004). This is one more important reason to continue breastfeeding.

Breastfeeding helps you interact more positively. Of all the laws we've described, skin-to-skin (chapter 2) is going to be the most helpful for you. Mothers who carry their babies by wearing them become more positive with them and more responsive to their cues. Also, having your baby near when you sleep is also going to be helpful, since you will be able to respond without being fully awake.

Get support. This is another time when you don't want to go it alone. It's important that you seek support from your partner, family, or friends. Support can lessen your depression and also help you be more positive with your baby. Try to find a local mothers' group or mother-to-mother breastfeeding group. Some moms have found that the women they meet in their childbirth education class can be a great source of support. And don't rule out online support. This is especially important where local in-person support is not available.

Most treatments for depression are compatible with breastfeeding. Getting help for your depression is going to benefit both you and your baby. Of the medications that are compatible with breastfeeding, Zoloft and Paxil have the best safety records (Hale 2004). The only ones that breastfeeding mothers should never take are called Monoamine Oxidase

Inhibitors (MAOIs), such as Nardil or Parnate. See our Web site for a full listing of your treatment options and how they impact breastfeeding.

DIFFICULT BIRTH

If you had a difficult birth, it could influence the ease with which you learn to breastfeed. These types of experiences can be physically and emotional difficult for women. Sometimes, the experiences are difficult enough that women become depressed or develop symptoms of post-traumatic stress disorder. On top of all that, women may also have trouble breastfeeding. But if breastfeeding is not going well, don't wait before you get some help. We've worked with enough women to tell you confidently that most of these problems are solvable, even if you've had a really difficult beginning.

There are three breastfeeding problems that seem to be more common following a difficult birth. These problems include delayed onset of lactation, temporary low milk supply, and breast refusal. All of these problems are discussed in more detail in other sections, so we'll mention them only briefly here.

Delayed onset of lactation. A highly stressful birth can delay when your milk increases. A study in Guatemala found that women who had high levels of the stress hormone cortisol after a difficult birth had a delay of several days (Grajeda and Perez-Escamilla 2002). Cesarean births can also delay when you first breastfeed. Although breastfeeding before the epidural wears off is most comfortable, not all mothers have this opportunity. Some mothers are not given their babies for several hours, or even overnight, after delivery (Rowe-Murray and Fisher 2002). But the good news is that this delay did not seem to have any long-term effects on mothers' ability to breastfeed or how long they breastfed.

Low milk supply. Researchers are starting to realize that the physiological aspects of a difficult birth can have an impact on breastfeeding. For example, severe postpartum hemorrhage can sometimes delay milk production. Low milk supply might occur if you were under severe stress during your labor and delivery, or had a mild to moderate postpartum hemorrhage (Willis and Livingstone 1995).

Breast refusal. Breastfeeding success is often even more important to mothers after a difficult birth than when birth goes smoothly. But related issues, such as separation of mother and baby and early supplementation, may cause difficulties. Sometimes a baby will respond to these difficulties by actively refusing her mother's breasts. Most mothers find this emotionally very difficult and often conclude that their babies do not like *them*. But this is definitely not the case (see below).

What to do if you are having problems. Fortunately, all these problems are solvable. But there are a few things that you must do.

- *Protect your milk supply.* If your baby is not breastfeeding well or is refusing the breast, you must protect your supply. That may mean renting a pump until things get back on track. You must remove milk from your breasts eight to twelve times a day to bring in a good supply. Law 4, "More breastfeeding at first means more milk later," is going to be helpful here, with a pump substituting for your baby.

- *Feed the baby.* If your milk supply is significantly lower than it should be, you may need to supplement with formula for a few days. While this is not ideal, it may be necessary. Keep your long-term goals in mind.

- *Have lots of contact with your baby.* Laws 1 and 2, using your baby's hardwiring and using skin-to-skin, are going to be especially relevant in your situation. Hold your baby and have lots of skin-to-skin contact. Allow your baby to practice breastfeeding when she is not particularly hungry but is in a quiet, alert state. Babies who are calm and not frantically hungry can, in most cases, be coaxed onto the breast. Make the breast a pleasant place to be.

- *Rule out physical trauma to the baby.* Sometimes after a difficult delivery, babies may be suffering from a birth-related injury. They may be sore from a vacuum extraction or forceps delivery. They may have a neck injury, broken collar bone (clavicle), or another physical issue. Being held in a certain way for breastfeeding may be painful. Watch your baby and see if that appears to be so. No one eats well when in pain, and adjustments may be necessary.

■ *Recognize the meaning of your baby's behavior.* If your baby is refusing the breast or not breastfeeding well, it doesn't mean she does not like breastfeeding—or you. While it is natural for mothers to sometimes feel that way, make the rational adult part of your brain keep repeating that it's simply not true. The more contact that you can have with your baby during this time, the better. Soon you will realize that your baby not only likes you, but actually prefers you to all other people.

If you are interested in more information, we refer you to an article on our Web site, "Making Peace with Your Birth Experience."

PAST SEXUAL ABUSE OR SEXUAL ASSAULT

For adult survivors of sexual abuse or assault, breastfeeding can also pose challenges. Unfortunately, sexual abuse and assault are relatively common experiences, affecting approximately 20 to 25 percent of women (Kendall-Tackett 2004). The reactions of abuse survivors to breastfeeding run the whole range of responses, from really disliking breastfeeding to finding it tremendously healing.

Interestingly, adult survivors are often interested in breastfeeding. Two studies have found that pregnant abuse survivors were more likely to say that they planned to breastfeed (Benedict, Paine, and Paine 1994) and were more likely to start breastfeeding in the hospital (Prentice et al. 2002) compared with nonabused women. If you are an abuse survivor who wants to breastfeed, we'd like to congratulate you for making a positive life choice to overcome your past and parent well.

We've included both sexual abuse and assault in this section because we have found that both can make a difference. Sexual abuse is often something that happens within the family and can include everything from fondling to rape. Sexual assault is often outside the family and can also include attacks by peers. We have found that women have similar reactions to both of these experiences.

If you are having a hard time with breastfeeding, we have some specific suggestions.

Figure out what makes you uncomfortable. Is it nighttime feeding? Is it your baby touching other parts of your body while nursing? Is it latching on? Or all of the above? The intense physical contact of breastfeeding may be very uncomfortable for you. You might find breastfeeding painful because your abuse experience lowered your pain threshold. The act of breastfeeding may also trigger flashbacks. There is a whole range of possible things that might be uncomfortable for you.

Can you address the problem? If skin-to-skin contact is bothering you, can you put a towel or cloth between you and the baby? Can you avoid the feedings that make you uncomfortable? Nighttime feedings are often a good candidate. Would you be more comfortable if you pumped and fed your baby with a bottle? Can you hold baby's other hand while breastfeeding to keep her from touching your body? Can you distract yourself while breastfeeding with TV or a book. (Many mothers have told us that this works well for them.) Experiment and find out what helps.

Remember that some breastfeeding is better than none. You may not be able to fully breastfeed, but every little bit helps. Even if you must pump milk and use a bottle; even if you are only breastfeeding once a day. Some abuse survivors find that they never love breastfeeding, but they learn to tolerate it. And that may be a more realistic goal for you.

Past abuse does not have to influence the rest of your life. We have both known many abuse survivors who have gone on to become wonderful mothers. We're confident that you can, too.

SPECIAL SITUATIONS: BABY

Babies may also have some physical challenges that influence their ability to breastfeed. These can be temporary, such as colds or the flu, or longer-term, such as prematurity, Down syndrome, or a cleft palate. In this section, we describe what to do when you need to temporarily stop breastfeeding, and how to bring in a full milk supply with a pump.

Acute or Chronic Health Problems

Sometimes even breastfed babies become sick. Or your baby may have a chronic health problem. In either case, as we explained in the introduction, the health outcomes of breastfeeding are better for you and your baby than using nonhuman milks. However, there may be some challenges. So here are suggestions on how to cope.

COLDS, FLU, OR EAR INFECTION

When your baby has a cold or the flu, she may not want to breastfeed. Breastfeeding may be difficult when she has a stuffy nose, because she can't breathe when she closes her mouth over your breast. Ear infections can also make her uncomfortable, especially when she is lying on her side. And the suction she creates to breastfeed can make her ears hurt. Even if uncomfortable, your milk is still the easiest food for her to handle, will better prevent dehydration, and will help her recover more quickly. Here are some strategies:

- Breastfeed your baby in a different position. Sometimes sitting up is more comfortable for babies with lots of congestion. Keep your baby upright at other times as well for better drainage.

- Breastfeed in a room with high humidity, either from a vaporizer or a running shower.

- Short, frequent feedings may be easier for your baby to manage.

- If your baby is very congested, contact her health-care provider for other suggestions.

If your baby is refusing to nurse, you need to express your milk and give it to her another way. Be sure to drain your breasts as often as you would have breastfed to keep up your milk supply and prevent mastitis. (See our upcoming section "When You Need to Temporarily Stop Breastfeeding.")

DIARRHEA, VOMITING, REFLUX DISEASE

Although it is less likely, breastfed babies sometimes develop these health problems. Breastfeeding is still your best approach.

Diarrhea. Diarrhea can develop from a variety of causes. Before assuming this is your baby's problem, first be sure that it is actual diarrhea and not simply the normal loose stools of a breastfed baby. It's real diarrhea if your baby has twelve to sixteen stools in a day, if the stools are watery with no substance, or if the stools suddenly seem a lot stinkier (normal stools of a breastfed baby have a mild scent). If your baby has green, frothy stools, refer to the section "Overabundant Milk Supply" in chapter 10 for strategies.

Continuing to breastfeed is the best thing you can do if your baby has diarrhea. This is true in all but some highly unusual situations (such as galactosemia, a rare metabolic disorder). In fact, although doctors used to tell mothers to wean temporarily when their babies had diarrhea, researchers have discovered that this is not helpful. You should be alert to signs of dehydration in a newborn, such as a weak cry, fewer than two wet diapers in a day, the fontanel (or soft spot on the head) looking sunken or depressed, dry eyes or mouth, and skin that stays pinched-looking after you gently pinch it. If you see these signs, contact your baby's doctor immediately.

Vomiting. Even healthy babies can spit up a lot of milk. If your baby is showing no other signs of illness, has at least three to four bowel movements a day (the size of a U.S. quarter, 2.5 cm, or larger), and is gaining weight well, this is no cause for concern. During the first four months, breastfed babies average a weight gain of about 6 ounces (170 g) a week. (This weight gain slows down as they get older.) If your baby is not gaining well, or if you are just concerned, contact your baby's healthcare provider. You might also try experimenting with smaller, more frequent breastfeedings to see if that cuts down on the amount of spit-up. Sometimes babies spit up because of mothers' desire to really "top off" their babies, or make them really full. This can also happen when a fast feeder is cajoled into breastfeeding longer, until the "right" number of minutes has passed. This extra milk has to go somewhere—in this case, back out.

If your baby is vomiting a lot because she is sick, you might try expressing some milk and letting your baby nurse on an almost-drained breast for comfort. That way, your baby will still get some milk and will have the comfort of breastfeeding. She may be able to tolerate smaller, frequent feedings better than the larger feedings that she is used to.

You do not have to wean or suspend breastfeeding when your baby is vomiting. This used to be the standard advice, but now research has demonstrated that this is not beneficial (Mohrbacher and Stock 2003). Unlike nonhuman milks, your milk is quickly and easily absorbed by your baby. You will want to watch for signs of dehydration (see above). If you see any, be sure to contact your baby's health-care provider immediately.

Reflux disease. Gastroesophageal reflux disease (GERD) is another health issue that can develop in the first year of life. Reflux occurs when stomach acid backs up into the esophagus, which is normal in all children and adults. However, when it damages these delicate tissues, it is considered a disease. Your baby may choke or cough while eating. Or she may arch back, turn her head, or flatten out, rather than cuddle and settle in when you try to feed her. She may have intense periods of crying during and after feedings. And finally, she may refuse to feed at all. All of these behaviors can be distressing to both you and your baby, but they are no reflection on you or your mothering skills. She is most likely in pain.

If you and your baby's health-care provider suspect reflux, you may decide on a trial of medication. If it helps, this can confirm reflux. There are also other strategies that can be helpful. Take advantage of gravity to keep your baby's stomach acid where it should be—in the stomach. To do this, always keep your baby's head higher than her bottom, and avoid bending your baby in the middle since this can also push on the stomach, making the acid rise.

A baby sling or carrier can be helpful to keep your baby upright. Use breastfeeding holds that keep your baby's head higher than her bottom. You may want to put a firm wedge under your baby to elevate her head while she sleeps. (But never use a pillow, as it's unsafe for your baby.) Sometimes mothers find that their babies sleep better in their car seats or bouncers. You might also find it helpful to elevate your baby's changing surface so her head is higher, and turn your baby side to side rather than bending her in the middle when changing diapers. Also, shorter, more frequent feedings may help your baby because her stomach won't be as full.

Two strategies that don't seem to work for babies with reflux are adding thickeners to their feedings and/or putting the baby on formula. Thickeners are unhelpful because they are introducing something other than human milk into the baby's immature gut. This can cause more problems than it solves. Also, if thickeners are mixed with human milk, the active enzymes in human milk break them down quickly. Similarly, using formula simply compounds your baby's problems since you are adding foreign proteins to your baby's system, which are harder to handle. Research indicates that babies with reflux do better on human milk than on formula, because human milk passes through the stomach faster, resulting in fewer symptoms (Mohrbacher and Stock 2003).

Prematurity, Down Syndrome, Cleft Lip or Palate

Another challenging situation some mothers face is having a baby who is physically compromised. Fortunately, even these babies can eventually breastfeed. And right from the start, your milk can make a difference in how healthy your baby is and when she can come home from the hospital.

PREMATURITY

Having a premature or low-birth-weight baby can be a very frightening experience. Premature babies can be low birth weight (3.3 to 5 lbs.; 1500 to 2500 g) or very low birth weight (less than 3.3 lbs.; 1500 g). You may be in shock after you've had your baby. Mothers often report feeling frightened, angry, guilty, and helpless. You may feel completely overwhelmed by the hospital environment and the emergency nature of your baby's birth. These feelings are normal. However, there are also some very important things that you can do to help your baby.

Your milk works like a medicine for your baby. Your body will produce exactly what your baby needs, starting with colostrum. As the mother of a premature baby, your milk is higher in anti-infective properties, nitrogen, protein nitrogen, sodium, chloride, iron, and fatty acids than mothers of full-term babies (Mohrbacher and Stock 2003). It also has even higher concentrations of those nonfood aspects of your milk that promote normal immune and digestive function than the milk of mothers of full-term babies. Your milk is just what your baby needs to grow and thrive. Research has found that preemies fed nonhuman milks have more life-threatening infections and lower intelligence as they mature (Mohrbacher and Stock 2003).

Protect your milk supply. Since premature babies can have difficulty breastfeeding, you will need to begin pumping immediately. Little babies sometimes tire easily and doze off before they have had enough to eat. Some cannot be brought to breast at all in the early weeks. Even if this is the case, they can be fed with your milk. See the final section in this chapter for instructions on how to establish a full milk supply with a pump.

Spend as much time as you can skin to skin with your baby. Fortunately, there have been some positive changes in the way that hospitals handle premature babies. In the bad old days, mothers were kept away from their babies until it was close to time for them to go home. Is it any wonder that mothers often felt disconnected from their babies and that it was necessary for "experts" to care for them?

In chapter 2, we described the importance of skin-to-skin contact in helping your baby grow and thrive. This simple technique increased the survival rate of premature babies in developing countries such as Colombia and South Africa. And it has been helpful in industrialized countries, as well. In one study, babies who were held skin to skin gained weight faster, had less stress, and went home sooner. These babies also were able to breastfeed sooner and skin-to-skin contact also increased their mothers' milk supply (Hurst 1997).

Skin-to-skin contact also increased mothers' feelings of confidence, decreased their sense of helplessness and depression, and helped mothers connect with their babies. Since you are protecting your milk supply by pumping, you can relax and enjoy your baby's initial attempts at breastfeeding, even if she isn't capable of fully feeding at the breast in the early days or weeks. Spending lots of time holding your baby can give you many opportunities to practice throughout the day. Review chapter 2 for more information, and check out the resources on our Web site (www.BreastfeedingMadeSimple.com).

Get support. Having a premature baby can be a difficult experience. Several recent studies have found that parents who have peer support feel less depressed and more confident as mothers (Kendall-Tackett 2005). Find out what sources of support are available locally or online. Reaching out to others can make a big difference in how well you cope and the ease of your transition into motherhood.

DOWN SYNDROME

Mothers of babies with Down syndrome can also suffer from shock and denial in the hours after their babies' births—especially if they didn't know before the baby was born. Babies with Down syndrome may also have some health issues, such as heart problems, that require immediate intervention. If so, they may need to be transferred to another hospital and be separated from you. This can be highly stressful for mothers who experience it. Fortunately, there are some steps that you can take to help you breastfeed your baby.

Your milk protects your baby. Since babies with Down syndrome are prone to respiratory infections and bowel problems, breastfeeding can help maintain good health. Even if you must pump in the beginning, your milk offers important protection.

Breastfeeding helps mouth and tongue coordination. Feeding your baby at the breast can help her gain better tongue control and can contribute to a more normal development of her facial muscles.

Skin-to-skin will help you and your baby. You might be concerned about how you will mother your baby. Skin-to-skin contact is a great place to start. It will increase your milk supply and help you tune in to your baby's cues. Review chapter 2 for more specific suggestions on skin-to-skin contact.

Offer your breast many times a day. Since babies with Down syndrome can be sleepy at the breast, you may find that your baby does better when she has short, frequent feedings throughout the day. If your baby is not gaining weight well, you may need to pump your hindmilk (the fattier milk at the end of the feeding) and give it to your baby in a bottle, supplementer, or other feeding device to make sure she gets enough calories.

Since babies with Down syndrome often have problems with tongue thrusting, it may be more challenging to get your baby latched on well. It may take a few extra tries, so you will want to start trying to latch your baby on before she is very hungry. Squeeze a few drops of milk onto your breast and encourage your baby to open wide.

Babies with Down syndrome also tend to have low muscle tone in their facial muscles. Because of this, they may need extra support when they are at the breast. Slide your fingers under your breast, forming a U. Slide your fingers forward so that your thumb and index finger are each on your baby's cheek (one on each side) to give her the extra support she needs to stay on the breast. Support your baby's chin at the bottom of the U. This is called the "Dancer Hand Position."

If your baby is choking while breastfeeding, position her so she is looking down at your nipple so that gravity will help slow milk flow. You can do this in a chair, leaning back. You can also add an extra pillow under your baby while leaning back slightly. This will tilt your breast upwards. Your baby may also need to be burped more often than a baby without Down syndrome if she is swallowing a lot of air when she nurses.

Breastfeeding is most definitely possible and desirable for the baby with Down syndrome. As your baby increases in muscle tone, breastfeeding will become easier and you'll be able to relax and enjoy the special closeness of the breastfeeding relationship.

CLEFT LIP OR PALATE

A "cleft" is an opening, and a cleft lip or palate refers to an opening in the lip or palate. These conditions can occur separately or together. If a baby has a cleft lip alone, this usually presents a more minor challenge to breastfeeding. Often all a mother needs to do is to use her thumb to plug the opening in the lip to maintain suction during breastfeedings. Cleft lips are usually surgically corrected at a young age, sometimes even right after birth.

But there are more serious feeding issues with a baby with a cleft palate. Until the opening is repaired, it can be challenging for your baby to feed either at the breast or with a bottle, because baby cannot create suction in the mouth to keep the breast or bottle in place. However, with patience and practice, at least partial breastfeeding is possible, and it is well worth the effort.

Your milk protects your baby. Because of the opening, babies with cleft palates are more prone to ear infections than babies without a cleft. Even partial human milk feedings can limit the number of infections your baby has and make her healthier overall. In addition, if your milk leaks into your baby's nose (which is a common problem for babies with a cleft palate), it will be much less irritating to these delicate tissues than formula.

Feeding at the breast can also help. Even if babies cannot fully feed at the breast, the act of breastfeeding helps their facial muscles develop normally. Feeding at the breast is also comforting in a way that bottle feeding is not. And babies with clefts often cannot use pacifiers.

In the lactation field, we used to be a lot more optimistic about whether babies with cleft palates could fully breastfeed. More recent research has indicated that full breastfeeding may be an elusive goal for all but a few. But partial breastfeeding and exclusive human milk feeding is entirely possible—especially if you work toward that goal from the beginning. Here are some things to try.

Pump to establish a full milk supply. Babies with a cleft palate are not able to drain the breast effectively, so think of the pump as your primary way of establishing a full milk supply and breastfeeding as an "extra." Give the pumped milk to your baby using another feeding method (see the upcoming section "Alternatives to Feeding at the Breast").

Try different positions. Experiment with different positions at the breast. Some will be more effective than others in allowing your breast to fill the gap and create the suction necessary to better drain your breast. For babies with a cleft lip, you may need to put a thumb or finger over the baby's top lip to create suction at the breast.

Support your baby's jaw. One technique you may find helpful is called the "Dancer Hand Position." Slide your fingers under your breast, forming a U. Your baby's chin should be at the bottom of the U. Slide your fingers forward so that your thumb and index finger are each on your baby's cheek (one on each side) to give her the extra support she needs to stay on the breast.

Use adaptive equipment. Some mothers have found it helpful to have a palatal obturator made for their baby. This is a special mouth appliance that can help babies feed more normally by providing a firm surface at the roof of the mouth. A Haberman feeder can also be helpful. This is a bottle designed for babies with feeding difficulties. The baby controls the milk flow with compression and it can be adjusted for a slower or faster flow.

Realize that feeding will take time. Whether feeding at the breast or with a bottle, feedings typically take two to three times longer for a baby with a cleft palate, so you should plan accordingly.

Breastfeed before and after surgery. At some point, your baby will have surgery to repair the cleft. Find out what your surgeon's guidelines are in terms of feeding before or after surgery. Most hospitals today allow breastfeeding up to four hours before surgery and as soon as a baby wakes from anesthesia. Refer your surgeon to *Breastfeeding: A Guide for the Medical Profession* (Lawrence and Lawrence 2005) if they have questions.

Tongue-Tie

If your baby has trouble breastfeeding, it may be because she has an abnormally short frenulum or a "tongue-tie." The frenulum is that stringy membrane under your baby's tongue. If that is tight, it can keep your baby's tongue from cupping under the breast and covering your baby's lower gum during feedings (you can have a helper check for this while you're breastfeeding). Possible indicators of this include:

- nipple pain or trauma despite a good latch-on;

- clicking sounds and/or difficulty staying on the breast;

- low weight gain.

If you suspect that this may be an issue for your baby, take a look at her tongue when her mouth is open. Babies with tongue-tie often have tongues that dip in the middle, forming a heart shape.

The treatment for tongue-tie is to clip the frenulum. That sounds much worse than it is for your baby. There are few nerves and blood vessels in that part of the body, and the procedure is usually done quickly in a doctor's office with no need for anesthesia. Your baby should be able to nurse immediately after the procedure. What you will notice is an amazing decrease in pain while your baby is at the breast. Oral surgeons, some dentists, pediatricians, or ear, nose, and throat specialists can perform this procedure. Ask around in your community. For more information, see the article on our Web site on tongue-tie. It has pictures and a good explanation of the procedure. Print this out and discuss it with your baby's doctor.

WHEN YOU NEED TO TEMPORARILY STOP BREASTFEEDING

If you need to temporarily stop breastfeeding because you or your baby are sick, or because you need to take a medication that is incompatible with breastfeeding, there are some steps that you can take to help both you and your baby.

Express your milk as many times per day as you would breast-feed. Your body is used to making milk in certain amounts. In order to maintain your supply, you will need to drain your breasts about as often as you would breastfeed. If you don't do this, you are at increased risk of engorgement and mastitis. Don't wait until your breasts feel full to start expressing your milk. Full breasts are a signal to your body to slow production (see chapter 6).

Use a good quality pump with double-pumping attachments. The best way to maintain your supply is with a rental pump or a single-user pump that provides at least forty to sixty suction-and-release cycles per minute. Other methods of breast draining may not be adequate unless you are very skilled at them.

Breastfeed long and often once you start again. If you find that you're not able to fit in enough pumpings, you might find that your supply is down. Once your baby is at the breast again, bring your supply back up with long, frequent breastfeedings. Use skin-to-skin contact and frequent feedings to reestablish your supply (see Laws 2 and 4). If low supply continues to be a problem, you might need to use an herb or medication to increase your supply (see "Low Milk Supply" in chapter

10). If your baby is refusing to breastfeed, see our section "Breast Refusal or Nursing Strike" in chapter 10 for suggestions.

ALTERNATIVES TO FEEDING AT THE BREAST

Even mothers who are breastfeeding sometimes need a way to feed their babies other than at the breast. Perhaps your baby is in the hospital and either tires quickly at the breast or is too small to breastfeed. Perhaps you need to return to work and your care provider needs to feed your baby. Perhaps you need to supplement your baby until your milk supply increases. Or maybe you are an adoptive mother and need to supplement as you build your own milk supply. Whatever the situation, you have a variety of options, including, of course, bottles. See chapter 9 for more information on using bottles.

If you're working with a lactation consultant, you may notice that he or she has some strong opinions about the "right" way to offer a supplemental feeding. Having worked with lots of mothers, we can tell you that there are many shades of gray when it comes to selecting a feeding method. What works well for one family is less effective for another. We encourage you to be flexible and see what works well for you.

The Methods

Although you may automatically think of a bottle, there are actually many ways to supplement a baby. If a baby is one month old or older and has been breastfeeding well, depending on circumstance, a bottle may be your best choice. If your baby is younger than a month and is not breastfeeding well, you might consider other options. The simplest is an ordinary spoon. Your baby can lick your milk or colostrum from the spoon. You can also use a small cup: one that you own (such as those that come on the top of children's liquid medications), or you can buy one that is specially designed to feed a baby. You can also use an eyedropper or feeding syringe. These allow you to slowly drip your breast milk or supplemental formula into your baby's mouth.

With each of these options, there are a few things to keep in mind.

- *Wait until your baby is alert and awake before trying to feed her.* Your baby needs to be awake enough to drink the milk you offer.

- *Swaddle or wrap your baby to keep her from bumping your feeding device.* Since it is much easier to spill, you will want to make sure that your baby's hands are not free.

- *Hold your baby upright while feeding.* Sitting up makes it easier for your baby to take the milk when ready.

- *Don't pour the milk into your baby's mouth.* Allow her to lick or sip it. That way, your baby can set the pace and not feel overwhelmed by the feeding. Don't offer more until your baby has had a chance to swallow.

The techniques we've described here are often most appropriate for newborns. Once your baby gets to be a few weeks or months old, you may find that your baby is less receptive to these approaches.

NURSING SUPPLEMENTER

Another option is a nursing supplementer. This is a device that includes a bottle or pouch that you wear around your neck that is filled with your milk or formula and thin tubing that leads from the container to your breast. When your baby latches on to your breast, she also takes the tubing. The supplement flows through the tubing while she is breastfeeding.

Supplementers may be used in a variety of situations, such as when your baby is premature, ill, or has a cleft palate. Your baby may be ill and have a weak suck, meaning she does not drain your breasts well enough for you to make enough milk. Your supply may be low after cutting back on breastfeeding or weaning. Or you may use a supplementer if you are nursing an adopted baby. While a supplementer can be a great solution for some mothers, others don't like it. Keep in mind that this is only one of your possible options. Talk with your local lactation consultant or your local hospital if you'd like to give this a try.

PUMPING TO ESTABLISH A FULL MILK SUPPLY

If for some reason your baby cannot breastfeed or is ineffective at the breast, you can bring in a full milk supply with a pump. Here are some suggestions to help you.

Start by pumping with a rental pump at least eight to ten times every twenty-four hours. This is as many times per day as your baby would be nursing. Use a double pumping kit to pump both breasts at once.

Pump at least ten to fifteen minutes per breast per pumping session. Do this for the first few days after birth until your milk comes in or increases. After that, as many times per day as you can fit it in, pump for two minutes after you see the last drop of milk, or up to thirty minutes total. Draining the breasts more fully increases your milk supply faster (see chapter 6). Do this until you have a full milk supply, ideally by day ten to fourteen.

Focus on the *number of pumpings per day,* not the time between pumpings. If you think in terms of the intervals between pumpings (for instance, every two or three hours), it is too easy for the number of pumpings to drop without your realizing it. Instead, when planning your day, think: "How can I fit in my ten or so pumpings?" If you can't pump during part of the day, pump every hour when you can to meet your goal.

Most women can cut back on the number of pumpings once they establish a full supply. The maximum amount of human milk a baby typically takes per day is 25 to 35 ounces (740 to 1035 ml). Your goal should be to pump this much milk within ten to fourteen days after birth, no matter how much your baby is taking. It may not be possible to increase to a full supply if you wait too long. Once you're pumping at least 25 to 35 ounces (740 to 1035 ml) a day, try cutting back to five to seven pumping sessions a day. Most women can maintain their supply at this level of pumping for as long as they choose. If your supply starts to decrease, this means you probably have a small breast storage capacity (see chapter 6), and you'll need to increase the number of pumpings to increase your supply.

Once you have a full supply, you may not need to pump during your normal sleeping hours. Until you have a full supply, pump at least once during the night and don't go longer than five hours between pumping sessions. Once you have a full supply, if your breast storage capacity is large enough, you may be able to pump right before bed and first thing in the morning without your milk supply dropping. If you can do this without discomfort, go ahead.

How to Wean from Pumping

If your baby is not breastfeeding and you are ready to wean from pumping, you can do it painlessly and safely using the same principles we described in chapter 7. Gradually cut back on pumping sessions by eliminating one daily pumping, give your body two to three days to adjust, and then eliminate another daily pumping. Repeat until you have eliminated all your pumping sessions, leaving the one before bedtime and the one when you get up for last. Another way is to stop pumping before you get as much milk as usual. For example, if you normally get 3 ounces (90 ml) at a pumping, stop at 2 ounces (60 ml) at each session. With either of these approaches (or a combination of both), if you feel full at any time, pump to comfort—not a full pumping, but long enough so that your breasts feel more comfortable. Leaving your breasts feeling full can cause pain and mastitis (see chapter 7). If your weaning is gradual enough, it should always be comfortable.

YOU'RE ON YOUR WAY

Having a baby is one of life's major transitions and learning to breastfeed can take patience and persistence, especially if you haven't had the chance to learn it by watching mothers breastfeed during your growing-up years. If your learning is just now beginning, you may need to review the information we shared with you many times as you get the hang of breastfeeding. We hope you find it helpful.

Also be sure to check out our Web site, www.Breastfeeding MadeSimple.com, which contains lots of information that just wouldn't fit in this book. It includes more details about special circumstances and much, much more.

You're most definitely on your way! Give your sweet baby a kiss for us. Your baby is very lucky you are learning what you need to know to make breastfeeding work. Many mothers think about the health effects of breastfeeding to help keep them motivated as they work their way through the early learning curve. What sometimes comes as a wonderful surprise, though, is the intimacy breastfeeding adds to their relationship with their baby. Breastfeeding is far more than food. It is also a way of giving and receiving love.

Enjoy the early weeks and months with your baby! This is truly one of life's special times.

Resources

FINDING SKILLED BREASTFEEDING HELP

Finding skilled help can be tricky, in part because there are different breastfeeding credentials reflecting different levels of education and training. Some of these initials, such as CLC, CLE, CBE, CBC, and LE, are awarded after attending a brief training course, usually less than one week long. A person with these initials may be helpful but may have limited skills and understanding and limited experience working one-on-one with breastfeeding mothers and babies.

On the other hand, the credential IBCLC indicates a level of basic competency (at the very least) in the field of lactation. These initials stand for "international board certified lactation consultant." To be awarded this credential, a person must pass an all-day certifying exam. But that is not all. To qualify to take that exam, she must first have a combination of formal education, breastfeeding education, and thousands of hours working one-on-one with breastfeeding mothers and babies. The following are some ways you can find an IBCLC:

- Check the registry on www.iblce.org. IBLCE is the International Board of Lactation Consultant Examiners, the organization that accredits lactation consultants. They have a complete list of IBCLCs all over the world.

- Click on "Find a Lactation Consultant" on www.ilca.org. ILCA is the International Lactation Consultant Association, the professional association for lactation consultants. Not all international board certified lactation consultants are members.

- Call your local hospital and ask to speak to the lactation consultant. Ask if she can help you or if she knows someone in your community who can.

- Check your telephone book under "Breastfeeding."

Another option is to contact a representative from a mother-to-mother breastfeeding group, such as La Leche League, Australian Breastfeeding Association, or Nursing Mothers Counsel. These women are volunteers who have breastfed their own children and have at least a basic understanding of breastfeeding. Some are highly skilled and some are relatively inexperienced. Ideally, if your problem is more complicated than they can help with or if you need to be seen and they are unable to do so, they will refer you to someone in your area who can provide the help you need.

To find your local representative, go online:

- La Leche League International—
www.lalecheleague.org

- Australian Breastfeeding Association—
www.breastfeeding.asn.au

- Nursing Mothers Counsel—www.nursingmothers.org

FINDING LOCAL SOURCES OF HELP

Doulas

"Doula" comes from the Greek word for servant and refers to someone who provides practical and emotional help to women before, during, and after birth.

www.dona.org—Doulas of North America (for labor-support doulas)

www.napcs.org—National Association of Postpartum Care Services (for postpartum doula care)

Breast Pumps, Rental or Purchase

To locate an Ameda rental pump or an Ameda Purely Yours purchase pump near you, contact Hollister, Inc., at 1-800-323-4060 (in the U.S.) or go online to www.hollister.com.

To locate a Medela rental pump or a Medela Pump In Style purchase pump near you, contact Medela, Inc., at 1-800- TELLYOU (in the U.S.) or go online to www.medela.com.

An Accurate Baby Scale

The BabyWeigh scale by Medela is available for rent and is accurate to 0.1 oz., making it reliable enough to measure the milk a baby takes at the breast. (Medela's Baby Checker scale is not accurate enough for this purpose.) To locate a BabyWeigh rental outlet near you, contact Medela at 1-800-TELLYOU or www.medela.com.

To Prevent Milk Leakage

To find LilyPadz, the silicone product that prevents milk leakage, go online to www.lilypadz.com.

WEB SITES OF INTEREST

www.BreastfeedingMadeSimple.com—Our Web site with lots of extras, including many additional links to relevant Web sites.

www.bfmed.org/protocol/cosleeping.pdf—Academy of Breastfeeding Medicine's Guidelines on Co-Sleeping and Breastfeeding.

www.nd.edu/~jmckenn1/lab/—Web site of James McKenna, researcher on parent/child co-sleeping.

www.bfar.org—Web site of Diana West, IBCLC. For women who are breastfeeding after breast reduction surgery.

RECOMMENDED BOOKS AND VIDEOS

Books

Hale, T. 2004. *Medications and Mothers' Milk*, 11th ed. Amarillo, TX.: Pharmasoft Publishing. Available from www.ibreastfeeding.com.

Kroeger, Mary, with Linda J. Smith. 2004. *Impact of Birthing Practices on Breastfeeding: Protecting the Mother and Baby Continuum*. Boston: Jones and Bartlett.

Palmer, Gabrielle. 1988. *The Politics of Breastfeeding*. London: Pandora.

West, Diana. 2001. *Defining Your Own Success: Breastfeeding After Breast Reduction Surgery*. Schaumburg, IL: La Leche League International.

Videos

Bergman, Nils. 2000. *Kangaroo Mother Care: Restoring the Original Paradigm for Infant Care and Breastfeeding*. This video is available at www.KangarooMotherCare.com.

Glover, Rebecca. 2002. *Follow Me Mum: The Key to Successful Breastfeeding*. Burswood, Western Australia: Tapestry Films. Available from http://www.rebeccaglover.com.au/ and www.ibreastfeeding.com.

References

Academy of Breastfeeding Medicine. 2003. *Clinical protocol number 6: Guidelines on co-sleeping and breastfeeding.* www.bfmed.org.

American Academy of Pediatrics Committee on Drugs (AAP). 2001. The transfer of drugs and other chemicals into human milk. *Pediatrics* 108:776-789.

American Academy of Pediatrics Subcommittee on Hyperbilirubinemia (AAP). 2004. Management of hyperbilirubinemia in the newborn infant 35 or more weeks of gestation. *Pediatrics* 114:297-316.

American Academy of Pediatrics Work Group on Breastfeeding (AAP). 2005. Breastfeeding and the use of human milk. *Pediatrics* 115:496-506.

American Psychiatric Association. 2000. *Diagnostic and Statistical Manual of Mental Disorders,* 4th ed., Text Revision. Washington, DC: Author.

Anisfeld, E., V. Casper, M. Nozyce, and N. Cunningham. 1990. Does infant carrying promote attachment? An experimental study of the effects of increased physical contact on the development of attachment. *Child Development* 61:1617-1627.

Armstrong, J., and J. Reilly. 2002. Breastfeeding and lowering the risk of childhood obesity. *Lancet* 359:2003-2004.

Azar, B. 2002. The postpartum cuddles: Inspired by hormones? *Monitor on Psychology* 33:9.

Bates, J., C. Maslin, and K. Frankel. 1985. Attachment security, mother-child interaction, and temperament as predictors of behavior problem ratings at three years. In *Growing Points in Attachment Theory and Research. Monographs of the Society for Research in Child Development*, edited by I. Bretherton and E. Waters. Chicago: Society for Research in Child Development.

Benedict, M., L. Paine, and L. Paine. 1994. *Long-term Effects of Child Sexual Abuse on Functioning in Pregnancy and Pregnancy Outcome.* Final report, National Center on Child Abuse and Neglect. Washington DC: National Center on Child Abuse and Neglect.

Benson, S. 2001. What is normal? A study of normal breastfeeding dyads during the first sixty hours of life. *Breastfeeding Review* 9:27-32.

Bergman, N. 2001. *Kangaroo Mother Care: Restoring the original paradigm for infant care and breastfeeding.* Presentation at La Leche League International's 29th Annual Seminar for Physicians on Breastfeeding, Chicago, IL.

————. 2001. *Kangaroo Mother Care: Restoring the original paradigm for infant care and breastfeeding.* Video available at www.Kangaroo MotherCare.com.

Bergman, N., and N. Jurisoo. 1994. The 'kangaroo-method' for treating low-birth-weight babies in a developing country. *Tropical Doctor* 24:57-60.

Bergman, N., L. Linley, and S. Fawcus. 2004. Randomized controlled trial of skin-to-skin contact from birth versus conventional incubator for physiological stabilization in 1200 to 2199 gram newborns. *Acta Paediatrica* 93:779-785.

Blumenthal, M., W. R. Busse, A. Goldberg, T. Hall, C. W. Riggins et al. eds. 1998. *The Complete German Commission E Monographs: Therapeutic Guide to Herbal Medicines*. Austin, TX: American Botanical Council.

Bumgarner, N. J. 2000. *Mothering Your Nursing Toddler*. Schaumburg, IL: La Leche League International.

Bushnell, J, F. Sai, and J. Mullin. 1989. Neonatal recognition of the mother's face. *British Journal of Developmental Psychology* 7:3-15.

Butte, N., et al. 2000. Infant feeding mode affects early growth and body composition. *Pediatrics* 106:1355-1366.

Cattaneo, A., et al. 1998. Kangaroo Mother Care for low birthweight infants: A randomized control trial in different settings. *Acta Paediatrica* 87:976-985.

Centers for Disease Control and Prevention. 2003. Breastfeeding practices: Results from the 2003 National Immunization Survey. http://www.cdc.gov/breastfeeding/NIS_data/age.htm.

Charpak, N., et al. 2001. A randomized controlled trial of Kangaroo Mother Care: Results of followup to 1 year corrected age. *Pediatrics* 108:1072-1079.

Chen, A., and W. Rogan. 2004. Breastfeeding and the risk of postneonatal death in the United States. *Pediatrics* 111:e435-e439.

Cregan, M., and P. Hartmann. 1999. Computerized breast measurement from conception to weaning: Clinical implications. *Journal of Human Lactation* 15:89-96.

Christensson K., et al. 1995. Separation distress call in the human neonate in the absence of maternal body contact. *Acta Paediatrica* 84:468-473.

Christensson, K., C. Siles, L. Moreno, et al. 1992. Temperature, metabolic adaptation and crying in healthy full term newborns cared for skin to skin or in a cot. *Acta Paediatrica* 81:488-493.

Combs, V., and S. Marino. 1993. A comparison of growth patterns in breast and bottle-fed infants with congenital heart disease. *Pediatric Nursing* 19:175-179.

Crockenberg, S., and K. McCluskey. 1986. Change in maternal behavior during the baby's first year of life. *Child Development* 57:746-753.

Cunningham, A., et al. 1991. Breast-feeding and health in the 1980s: A global epidemiologic review. *Journal of Pediatrics* 118:1-8.

Daly, S., and P. Hartmann. 1995. Infant demand and milk supply. Part 2: The short-term control of milk synthesis in lactating women. *Journal of Human Lactation* 11:27-37.

Daly, S., et al. 1993. The short-term synthesis and infant-regulated removal of milk in lactating women. *Experimental Physiology* 78:209-220.

deCarvalho, M., et al. 1984. Does the duration and frequency of early breastfeeding affect nipple pain? *Birth* 11:81-84.

DeMarzo, S., J. Seacat, and M. Neifert. 1991. Initial weight loss and return to birth weight criteria for breast-fed infants: Challenging the "rules of thumb." *American Journal of the Diseases of Children* 145:402.

Dettwyler, K. 1995. A time to wean: The hominid blueprint for the natural age of weaning in modern human populations. In *Breastfeeding: Biocultural Perspectives*, edited by P. Stuart-Macadam and K. Dettwyler. New York: Aldine de Gryter.

Dodd, V., and C. Chalmers. 2003. Comparing the use of hydrogel dressings to lanolin ointment with lactating mothers. *Journal of Obstetric, Gynecologic, and Neonatal Nursing* 32:486-494.

Dombrowski, M. A., G. C. Anderson, and C. Santori. 2001. Kangaroo (skin-to-skin) care with a postpartum woman who felt depressed. *Maternal Child Nursing* 26:214-215.

Duncan, B., et al. 1993. Exclusive breast-feeding for at least 4 months protects against otitis media. *Pediatrics* 91:867-872.

Dunham, C. 1992. *Mamatoto: A celebration of birth*. New York: Viking Penguin.

Dusdieker, L., et al. 1985. Effect of supplemental fluids on human milk production. *Journal of Pediatrics* 106:207-211.

Eisenberg, A., S. Hathaway, and H. Murkoff. 2003. *What to Expect the First Year*. 2nd ed. New York: Workman Publishing Company.

Feldman, R., et al. 2004. Mother-child touch patterns in infant feeding disorders: Relation to maternal, child, and environmental factors. *Journal of the American Academy of Child and Adolescent Psychiatry* 43:1089-1097.

Feldman, R., et al. 2002. Skin-to-skin contact (Kangaroo Care) promotes self-regulation in premature infants: Sleep-wake cyclicity, arousal modulation and sustained exploration. *Developmental Psychology* 38:194-197.

Feldman, R., et al. 1999. The nature of the mother's tie to her infant: Maternal bonding under conditions of proximity, separation, and potential loss. *Journal of Child Psychology and Psychiatry* 40:929-939.

Fifer, W., and C. Moon. 1994. The role of the mother's voice in the organization of brain function in the newborn. *Acta Paediatrica Supplementum* 397:86-93.

Freed, G. L., S. J. Clark, J. A. Lohr, and J. R. Sorenson. 1995a. Pediatrician involvement in breastfeeding promotion: A national study of residents and practitioners. *Pediatrics* 96:490-494.

Freed, G. L., S. J. Clark, J. R. Sorenson, J. A. Lohr, R. Cefalo, and P. Curtis. 1995b. National assessment of physicians' breastfeeding knowledge, attitudes, training, and experience. *Journal of the American Medical Association* 273:472-476.

Glover, R. 2002. *Follow Me Mum: The Key to Successful Breastfeeding*. Burswood, Western Australia: Tapestry Films.

———. 2004. Lessons from innate feeding abilities. Presentation at the International Lactation Consultant Association, Scottsdale, AZ.

Goldman, A., et al. 1983. Immunologic components in human milk during the second year of lactation. *Acta Paediatrica Scandinavia* 72:461-462.

Grajeda, R., and R. Perez-Escamilla. 2002. Stress during labor and delivery is associated with delayed onset of lactation among urban Guatemalan women. *Journal of Nutrition* 132:3055-3060.

Gray, L., L. Watt, and E. Blass. 2000. Skin-to-skin contact is analgesic in healthy newborns. *Pediatrics* 105:e14-e20.

Gulick, E. 1986. The effects of breastfeeding on toddler health. *Pediatric Nursing* 12:51-54.

Hale, T. 2004. *Medications and Mothers' Milk*, 11th ed. Amarillo, TX: Pharmasoft Publishing.

Harlow, H. F. 1959. The nature of love. *American Psychologist* 13:573-685.

Hanson, L. 2004. *Immunobiology of Human Milk: How Human Milk Protects Infants.* Amarillo, TX: Pharmasoft Publishing.

Hausman, B. 2003. A formal look at formula promotion. Presentation at the International Lactation Consultant Association, Sydney, Australia.

Heinrichs, M., I. Newmann, and E. Ulriket. 2002. Lactation and stress: Protective effects of breast-feeding in humans. *Stress* 5:195-203.

Helm, A. August 15, 2004 post on Lactnet, lactation professional listserv. Reprinted with permission.

Hillervik-Lindquist, C., et al. 1991. Studies on perceived breast milk insufficiency: III. Consequences for breast milk consumption and growth. *Acta Paediatrica Scandanavia* 80:297-303.

Holliday, K., et al. 1991. Growth of human milk-fed and formula-fed infants with cystic fibrosis. *Journal of Pediatrics* 118:77-79.

Høst, A. 1991. Importance of the first meal on the development of cow's milk allergy and intolerance. *Allergy Proceedings* 12:227-232.

Humphrey, S. 2003. *The Nursing Mother's Herbal.* Minneapolis: Fairview Press.

Hurst, N., et al. 1997. Skin-to-skin holding in the neonatal intensive care unit influences maternal milk volumes. *Journal of Perinatology* 17:213-217.

Illingsworth, P. et al. 1986. Diminution in energy expenditure during lactation. *British Medical Journal* 292:437-440.

Johnston, C., et al. 2003. Kangaroo Care is effective in diminishing pain response in preterm neonates. *Archives of Pediatric and Adolescent Medicine* 157:1084-1088.

Jones, G., et al. 2003. How many child deaths can we prevent this year? *Lancet* 362:65-71.

Jones, N. A., B. A. McFall, and M. A. Diego. 2004. Patterns of brain electical activity in infants of depressed mothers who breastfeed and bottle-feed: The mediating role of infant temperament. *Biological Psychology* 67:103-124.

Keane, V., et al. 1988. Do solids help baby sleep through the night? *American Journal of the Diseases of Childhood* 142:404-405.

Kearney, M., and L. Cronenwett. 1991. Breastfeeding and employment. *Journal of Obstetric, Gynecologic, and Neonatal Nursing* 20:471-480.

Kendall-Tackett, K. A. 2004. *Breastfeeding and the Sexual Abuse Survivor.* Lactation Consultant Series 2, Unit 9. Schaumburg, IL: La Leche League International.

————. 2005. *Depression in New Mothers: Causes, Consequences, and Treatment Options.* Binghamton, NY: Haworth Press.

Kendall-Tackett, K. A., and M. Sugarman. 1995. The social consequences of long-term breastfeeding. *Journal of Human Lactation* 11:179-183.

Klaus, M., and P. Klaus. 2000. *Your Amazing Newborn.* New York: Perseus Books.

Konner, M. 1976. Maternal care, infant behavior and development among the !Kung. In *Kalahari Hunter-gatherers: Studies of the !Kung San and Their Neighbors,* edited by R. B. Lee and I. DeVore. Cambridge, MA: Harvard University Press.

Kramer, M., et al. 2001. Promotion of breastfeeding intervention trial. *Journal of the American Medical Association* 85:413-420.

Kroeger, M., with L. J. Smith. 2004. *Impact of Birthing Practices on Breastfeeding: Protecting the Mother and Baby Continuum.* Boston: Jones and Bartlett.

Labbok, M., et al. 2004. Breastfeeding: Maintaining an irreplaceable immunological resource. *Nature Reviews/Immunology* 4:565-573.

Lawrence, R., and R. Lawrence. 2005. *Breastfeeding: A Guide for the Medical Profession.* St. Louis, MO: Elsevier Mosby.

Macknin, M., et al. 1989. Infant sleep and bedtime cereal. *American Journal of the Diseases of Childhood* 143:1066-1068.

Matthieson, A., A. Ransjö-Arvidson, E. Nissen, and K. Uvnäs-Moberg. 2001. Postpartum maternal oxytocin release by newborns: Effects of infant hand massage and sucking. *Birth* 28:13-19.

Mead, M., and N. Newton. 1967. Cultural patterns of perinatal behavior. In *Childbearing: Its Social and Psychological Aspects*, edited by S. Richardson and A. Guttmacher. Baltimore: Williams & Wilkins.

Mezzacappa, E. S., and E. S. Katkin. 2002. Breastfeeding is associated with reduced perceived stress and negative mood in mothers. *Health Psychology* 21:187-193.

Michelsson K., et al. 1996. Crying in separated and non-separated newborns: Sound spectrographic analysis. *Acta Paediatrica* 85:471-475.

Mikiel-Kostyra, K., J. Mazur, and I. Boltruszko. 2002. Effect of early skin to skin contact after delivery on duration of breastfeeding: A prospective cohort study. *Acta Paediatrica* 91:1301-1367.

Milligan, R., et al. 1996. Positioning intervention to minimize fatigue in breastfeeding women. *Applied Nursing Research* 9:67-70.

Mitoulas, L., et al. 2002. Efficacy of breast milk expression using an electric breast pump. *Journal of Human Lactation* 18:344-351.

Mohrbacher, N. 1993. How often should a baby breastfeed? *BabyTalk,* September, 40-41.

———. 1995. *Approaches to Weaning.* Publication No. 307-17. Schaumburg, IL: LaLeche League International.

Mohrbacher, N., and J. Stock. 2003. *The Breastfeeding Answer Book.* Schaumburg, IL: La Leche League International.

Molbak, K., et al. 1994. Prolonged breastfeeding, diarrhoeal disease, and survival of children in Guinea-Bissau. *British Medical Journal* 308:1403-1406.

Montagu, A. 1978. *Touching: The Human Significance of the Skin.* New York: Harper & Row.

Mortensen, E., et al. 2002. The association between duration of breast-feeding and adult intelligence. *JAMA* 287:2365-2371.

Nehlig, A., and G. Debry. 1994. Consequences on the newborn of chronic maternal coffee during gestation and lactation: A review. *Journal of the American College of Nutrition* 13:6-21.

Neville, M., et al. 1988. Studies in human lactation: Milk volumes in lactating women during onset of lactation and full lactation. *American Journal of Clinical Nutrition* 48:1375-1386.

Newman, J., and T. Pitman. 2000. *The Ultimate Breastfeeding Book of Answers.* Roseville, CA: Prima.

Newton, N. 1978. The role of oxytocin reflexes in three interpersonal reproductive acts: Coitus, birth, and breastfeeding. *Clinical Psychoneuroendocrinology in Reproduction* 22:411-418.

Polan, H. J., and M. Ward. 1994. Role of the mother's touch in failure to thrive: A preliminary investigation. *Journal of the American Academy of Child and Adolescent Psychiatry* 33:1098-1105.

Prentice, A., et al. 1989. Evidence for local feedback control of human milk secretion. *Biochemical Society Transactions* 17:489-492.

Prentice, A., et al. 1983. Dietary supplementation of lactating Gambian women. I. Effect on breast milk volume and quality. *Human Nutrition: Clinical Nutrition* 37C:53-64.

Prentice, J. C., M. C. Lu, L. Lange, and N. Halfon. 2002. The association between reported childhood sexual abuse and breastfeeding initiation. *Journal of Human Lactation* 18:219-226.

Quillin, S., and L. L. Glenn. 2004. Interaction between feeding method and co-sleeping on maternal-newborn sleep. *Journal of Obstetric, Gynecologic, and Neonatal Nursing* 33:580-588.

Ramsay, D., et al. 2004. Ultrasound imaging of milk ejection in the breast of lactating women. *Pediatrics* 113:361-367.

Ransjö-Arvidson, A., et al. 2001. Maternal analgesia during labor disturbs newborn behavior: Effects on breastfeeding, temperature, and crying. *Birth* 28:5-12.

Renfrew, M., C. Fisher, and S. Arms. 2004. *Bestfeeding: How to Breastfeed Your Baby*. Berkeley, CA: Celestial Arts.

Righard, L. 1998. Are breastfeeding problems related to incorrect breastfeeding technique and the use of pacifiers and bottles? *Birth* 25:40-44.

Righard, L., and M. Alade. 1990. Effect of delivery room routines on success of first breast feed. *Lancet* 336:1105-1107.

————. 1992. Sucking technique and its effect on success of breastfeeding. *Birth* 19(4):185-193.

Riva, E., et al. 1996. Early breastfeeding is linked to higher intelligence quotient scores in dietary treated phenylketonuric children. *Acta Paediatrica* 85:56-58.

Rogers, C., et al. 1987. Weaning from the breast: Influences on maternal decisions. *Pediatric Nursing* 13:341-345.

Rowe-Murray, H. J., and J. R. W. Fisher. 2002. Baby friendly hospital practices: Cesarean section is a persistent barrier to early initiation of breastfeeding. *Birth* 29:124-131.

Royal College of Midwives. 2002. *Successful Breastfeeding*. London: Churchill Livingstone.

Schulte, P. 1995. Minimizing alcohol exposure of the breastfeeding infant. *Journal of Human Lactation* 11:317-319.

Seammon, R. E., and L. Q. Doyle. 1920. Observations on the capacity of the stomach in the first ten days of postnatal life. *American Journal of the Diseases of Children* 20:516-538.

Sepkoski, C., et al. 1992. The effects of maternal epidural anesthesia on neonatal behavior during the first month. *Developmental Medicine and Child Neurology* 34:1072-1080.

Shrago, L. 1998. Adequacy of breastmilk intake: Assessment and interventions. Presentation at the La Leche League International Lactation Consultant Workshop, Chicago, IL.

Smillie, C. 2004. Baby-led latching: A neurobehavioral approach. Presentation at Wisconsin Association of Lactation Consultants, Appleton, WI.

Stern, G., and L. Kruckman. 1983. Multi-disciplinary perspectives on postpartum depression: An anthropological critique. *Social Science and Medicine* 17:1027-1041.

Sugarman, M., and K. A. Kendall-Tackett. 1995. Weaning ages in a sample of American women who practice extended breastfeeding. *Clinical Pediatrics* 34:642-647.

Taylor, S. E., et al. 2000. Biobehavioral responses to stress in females: Tend-and-befriend, not fight-or-flight. *Psychological Review* 107:411-429.

Törnhage, C-J., et al. 1999. First week Kangaroo Care in sick, very preterm infants. *Acta Paediatrica* 88:1402-1404.

Toschke, A. M., et al. 2002. Overweight and obesity in 6 to 14 year old Czech children in 1991: Protective effect of breastfeeding. *Journal of Pediatrics* 141:764-769.

Uvnäs-Moberg, K. 1998. Oxytocin may mediate the benefits of positive social interaction and emotions. *Psychoneuroendocrinology* 23:819-835.

Uvnäs-Moberg, K., et al. 1987. Release of GI hormones in mothers and infants by sensory stimulation. *Acta Paediatrica Scandanavia* 76:851-860.

Weetman, A. P. 1997. Fortnightly review: Hypothyroidism: Screening and subclinical disease. *British Medical Journal* 314:1175-1178.

West, D. 2001. *Defining Your Own Success: Breastfeeding After Breast Reduction Surgery*. Schaumburg, IL: La Leche League International.

Wiessinger, D. 1998. A breastfeeding tool using a sandwich analogy for latch-on. *Journal of Human Lactation* 14:51-56.

Willis, C., and V. Livingstone. 1995. Infant insufficient milk syndrome associated with maternal postpartum hemorrhage. *Journal of Human Lactation* 11:123-126.

Woodbury, R. M. 1925. *Infant Mortality and Its Causes.* Baltimore: Williams & Wilkins.

Woolridge, M., and C. Fisher. 1988. Colic, "overfeeding," and symptoms of lactose malabsorption in the breast-fed baby: A possible artifact of feed management? *Lancet* 2 (8605): 382-384.

World Health Organization (WHO). 2001. *The Optimal Duration of Exclusive Breastfeeding: Report of an Expert Consultation.* Geneva, Switzerland: Author.

Yamauchi, Y., and I. Yamanouchi. 1990. Breast-feeding frequency during the first 24 hours after birth in full-term neonates. *Pediatrics* 82:171-175.

Zangen, S., et al. 2001. Rapid maturation of gastric relaxation in newborn infants. *Pediatric Research* 50:629-632.

Zeskind, P., and D. Goff. 1992. Rhythmic organization of heart rate in breast-fed and bottle-fed newborn infants. *Early Development and Parenting* 1:79-87.

Nancy Mohrbacher, IBCLC, is an international board-certified lactation consultant who has worked extensively with breastfeeding families for more than twenty years. She is coauthor of *The Breastfeeding Answer Book*, a research-based guide for lactation professionals, and currently works as lactation education specialist at Hollister, Incorporated, maker of the Ameda breast pumps. She has contributed regularly to *BabyTalk* magazine and many other publications.

Kathleen Kendall-Tackett, Ph.D., IBCLC, is a health psychologist and international board-certified lactation consultant. She is research associate professor of psychology at the University of New Hampshire's Family Research Lab in Durham, NH, and a member of La Leche League International's board of directors. She is author or editor of eleven books, including *The Hidden Feelings of Motherhood* and *Depression in New Mothers*.

Foreword writer Jack Newman, MD, is a pediatrician and coauthor of *The Ultimate Breastfeeding Book of Answers*.

Some Other
New Harbinger Titles

Helping A Child with Nonverbal Learning Disorder, 2nd edition,
　　Item 5266 $15.95

The Introvert & Extrovert in Love, Item 4863 $14.95

The Estrogen-Depression Connection, Item 4832 $16.95

The Feel-Good Guide to Fibromyalgia & Chronic Fatigue Syndrome,
　　Item 4894 $14.95

Watercooler Wisdom, Item 4364 $14.95

The Juicy Tomato Guide to Ripe Living After 50, Item 4321 $16.95

What's Right With Me, Item 4429 $16.95

The Balanced Mom, Item 4534 $14.95

Women Who Worry Too Much, Item 4127 $13.95

In Harm's Way, Item 4003 $14.95

Breastfeeding Made Simple, Item 4046 $16.95

The Well-Ordered Office, Item 3856 $13.95

Talk to Me, Item 3317 $12.95

Romantic Intelligence, Item 3309 $15.95

Transformational Divorce, Item 3414 $13.95

The Rape Recovery Handbook, Item 3376 $15.95

Eating Mindfully, Item 3503 $13.95

Sex Talk, Item 2868 $12.95

Everyday Adventures for the Soul, Item 2981 $11.95

A Woman's Addiction Workbook, Item 2973 $19.95

The Daughter-In-Law's Survival Guide, Item 2817 $12.95

PMDD, Item 2833 $13.95

The Vulvodynia Survival Guide, Item 2914 $16.95

Love Tune-Ups, Item 2744 $10.95

Brave New You, Item 2590 $13.95

The Woman's Book of Sleep, Item 2418 $14.95

Call **toll free, 1-800-748-6273,** or log on to our online bookstore at **www.newharbinger.com** to order. Have your Visa or Mastercard number ready. Or send a check for the titles you want to New Harbinger Publications, Inc., 5674 Shattuck Ave., Oakland, CA 94609. Include $4.50 for the first book and 75¢ for each additional book, to cover shipping and handling. (California residents please include appropriate sales tax.) Allow two to five weeks for delivery.

Prices subject to change without notice.